I dedicate this book to my husband Eric and my sons Zack, Clay and Troy. They are the reasons I am a Survivor. They are my lifelines. Love, Peace, Strength, Hope and Courage.

In memory of Auntie Marguerite

I honor all breast cancer survivors with my words and my story, Namaste.

INTRODUCTION

"Mrs. Taranto, we've found a small cancer". I heard the words as I stood in my kitchen, alone on Thursday afternoon, May 4, 2006. My legs turned to wet noodles, caterpillars gave birth to butterflies in my stomach and my head was suddenly on some very rough seas without motion medication. In December of 2005 I visited my primary physician for my yearly physical. She ran the usual blood work on me, checked my vitals, performed a manual breast exam, discussed family history, and set a date for my mammogram. She also made an appointment for me to undergo a breast MRI, because of the history of breast cancer in my family. My maternal aunt succumbed to the horrible epidemic in 1995 and my maternal grandmother was a long time sufferer of uterine cancer that spread to her lungs. Suffice it to say, my mammogram came back completely normal. I was relieved. I decided (being the self-diagnostician that I am) to cancel my MRI. I determined that a clean mammogram was all the proof I needed that I was free of cancer. I was never so wrong. After 5 months of prolonging the inevitable, I underwent my breast MRI May 1, 2006. "Mrs. Taranto, we've found a small cancer" were the words I will never forget. The world stopped and I felt desperately alone. On May 4, 2006 Dr. Alan Semine uttered that sentence to me which seemed surreal...but it wasn't. It was VERY real.

Then I asked the news breaking doctor to repeat what he had told me. He did, and the room went gray. I was scanned, poked, prodded, x-rayed, and biopsied for the 3 days leading up to this phone call. I, not even for a moment, considered a positive result. My annual mammogram was clean in December. What didn't it show? It didn't show what a mammogram never would. I had invasive lobular carcinoma...breast cancer. This type of breast cancer cannot be seen on a mammogram, ever. Thank God my primary physician, Dr. Jill, ordered a breast MRI in conjunction with the mammogram because of my family history. I should have gone when it was originally scheduled but here I was in May getting my 1st breast MRI so I didn't know what to expect. I certainly didn't anticipate lying face down on a slab with two holes where

4

my breasts would dangle while I went blindly, waist deep, into a tunnel. I felt like there should be a farmer underneath me milking my breasts like udders! I counted backwards from the time limit the technician cited to me in seconds for each scan. This calmed my overactive nerves and sped up the time in my mind. The clanking noises are scary and the solitude in that tunnel, for me, was almost unbearable. I regretted, in spades, not taking my clonazepam beforehand. After about 45 minutes with a midway dye injection it was over. Now I had to wait for the doctor to call me. That was a Monday. Tuesday Dr. Jill actually called me and said the MRI showed something suspicious. The chief of radiology was in charge of my case and happened to know Dr. Jill. She said I needed to get up to the hospital for a biopsy of the suspicious area. Eric drove me, stayed with me during the procedure, and agreed with me on the way home that it'd turn out to be inflammation or a cyst or any number of other possibilities. For once in my life I truly wasn't worried. Thursday, May 4th, the phone call came. BOOM...

Ok. Now what? My emotions went into overdrive. I was nervous, surprised, alarmed, overwhelmed, and angry. My life as a mom of 3 growing boys was about to be seriously disrupted. I called my husband, Eric, at work. He, like me, never suspected the worst. He was confident that I'd be just fine. We decided it'd be best if he came home because concentrating at his work was not an option anymore. Plus, we could sense over the phone that we needed to be together. I called my cousin, a breast cancer survivor. Then I called Will. Will's surname is Power and I needed him to release this life altering news to my boys, my siblings and my parents. I invited some calm into the room, got my sweatshirt on and went to my son Zack's lacrosse game. The terrorist inside me was weighing heavily on my brain, but at that moment, to me, being a bleacher mom was more important. Eric left work and met me in the stands and to my surprise, my cousin and one of my best friends did too. The sun radiated just the right amount of heat over the field, but I was chilled to the bone. My cousin and my friend cried and hugged me but I felt a strange sense of distance to them. Their emotions were affirmation of my cancer and I wanted to cognitively run away from it. I all but ignored them and focused on the game. We lost. I made an appointment with Dr. Jill for the next day. She's been my primary physician since 1997. I needed her input on the best medical care possible, and trusted her implicitly.

 That night at dinner we played a game called 'high/low'. Each person speaks of the highest moment in their day, and the lowest. This is how we decided to tell the boys about my breast cancer. They were 16, 14, and 9, or about to be, at the time of my diagnosis. I didn't anticipate any specific reaction from any of the boys because we'd never experienced this type of crisis, ever. Suddenly I was in the company of young men. When it was my turn, I told them watching Zack's lacrosse game in the warm sun was my high point and the phone call from my radiologist was the lowest point of my day. I told my babies I had breast cancer. I told them I wouldn't ask 'why me', and that they shouldn't either. Cancer isn't picky. It just picks. It took several minutes to settle in, but settle in it did. They realized, as Eric and I already had, that their lives were no longer the same. They were young boys. They didn't want to know the particulars. They just wanted to know that I'd get through this and still be 'mom'. Their positive outlook, willingness to fight, inquisitive demeanor and a host of other characteristics was my source of strength. My sons convinced me that I had staying power with their retort. My new identity was about to be introduced to everyone...Noreen (or Noah), breast cancer survivor.

CHAPTER ONE

The next morning, Friday, May 5th, I worked, came home midafternoon, and then readied myself to see Dr. Jill. Coincidentally, Clay, my middle son, and I were attending a Red Sox game that night, so he agreed to accompany me to my appointment and we could continue on to Boston right after. He was 14. This was one of those moments when you wonder as a mom if you're making the right decision. I was quite guarded until now, and was wearing a coat of 'don't lose it' armor around my boys. I didn't want Clay to be witness to my armor cracking. We pulled into the medical building and, surprise, my friend Lynn was waiting for me! Lynn is the aforementioned friend who met me at Lacrosse with my cousin. Our families had met in 1992 when we moved to Mansfield MA, on the same street. Our older boys, Zack and Michael would go on to be best friends, even attend college together as roommates, and graduate in December, 2012! We shared most holidays together, travelled together, did all the kids' sports stuff together, and so much more. Lynn's mom is a breast cancer survivor. Lynn shared with me that she was worried how sedate I was being, and wanted to hear what Dr. Jill's recommendations were. She was acutely aware of my ongoing and ever present struggle with anxiety, and since I wasn't displaying any, she was nervous. Dr. Jill said she could send me into Boston, Dana Farber, Brigham and Women's, etc., but that knowing me, I'd get rattled by the commute, especially if not feeling well. She also said that though the physicians in Boston are among the best in their prospective fields, because of that they are often called away. She knew I'd need consistency and that my youngest was born at Newton/Wellesley hospital, where my cancer was detected, and is an easy ride. She helped me arrange a meeting there for the following Thursday. The Sox won...FLUTTER.

Sunday, May 7th, 2006 was my next hurdle. It also happened to be Clay's birthday. My parents were hosting a family gathering at their home in Marshfield MA, a picturesque beach town that some call the Irish Riviera! My cousins, their families, aunts, uncles and my brother and his family were there. I have two sisters.

One lives in Pittsburgh with her family and the other was on a trip to Disney with her family. I had to call Cara and tell her over the phone because I wouldn't see her until July when we planned a trip to PA for the 4th. She crumbled. Cara is the middle sister, our redheaded firecracker! She is an accomplished gymnastics coach, a formidable gourmet cook, a gracious hostess, an allegiant friend, a devoted mom to Jarrett and Bryer, and wife to Bill, my wonderfully jocular brother-in-law. Cara is also Little Niagra when presented with ANY daunting news relative to her family, but she quickly clears out the cobwebs, shifts into auto pilot, and confronts the situation. I knew, though distance separated us, she was a saving grace to have on my team. Julie, my youngest baby sister lived in the next town so I decided to wait until she got home from vacation and tell her in person, in a hug. The hardest part for me in all of this was that I wanted to make sure my family was emotionally upright to withstand what was about to break and enter our lives. I'm the oldest of 4. I feel an intrinsic responsibility to my younger siblings. I'm the protector, at least from my perspective. I'm the big sister and though Kenan, my brother is the 'go to' guy in our family, I work out hard to keep my shoulders strong for leaning. That's not to say we didn't all turn to each other in times of crisis or tragedy, we did, and do. When our nana died 7/12/1994 our hearts were shattered and none of us was stronger or weaker than the other. We dove in the deep end of sadness together. Well, the hierarchy tables were about to be turned.

14

I waited for most of my extended family to leave my parent's before I dropped the proverbial bomb. Kenan was outside with his wife Shelby and my 2 nieces. I always knew Kenan to be a 'guy's guy', tough as nails, a rock. He also has this billowy soft spot for his family. He's weathered many storms, both physically and professionally but somehow I knew that my news would sting. I was right. I leaned on his jeep, asked them all to join hands, and stung them, deep. They cried. I, surprisingly, did not. I maintained my compelling need to nurture and my mask of confidence, and informed them what my upcoming weeks would require. It was a few days later when I received am extremely personal, heartfelt depiction of what each of my siblings have endured, and overcome from Kenan. He outlined defeat of birth defects, lung disease, property loss due to fire, anxiety disorder, unexpected death and other imposing obstacles our family had faced. He confidently expressed, through words, that I'd overcome this obstacle facing me, with all of my family's support. We stayed outside, breathing in the salty sea air, until the inevitable was upon me. I needed to tell my mom and dad I had breast cancer...UGH.

My mom's sister, Marguerite, battled breast cancer for 10 years before she died. My uncle Charlie, Marguerite's husband, his new wife Carol, and my cousin Dee, Marguerite's daughter, were still at the party. I decided to share my news with Dee privately, before telling her dad or my folks. When I sat down with her on the sun porch, I reached for her hands and cupped them in mine. She looked at me knowingly, nodded her head, and hugged me. I didn't have to utter a word. She just knew. Dee asked me more details, but I remember being too preoccupied with how to tell my parents to answer most of her questions. I promised her I'd call her later. We went in to the living room. Mom and Dad were seated together on their loveseat so I planted myself on the arm and simply engaged in the ongoing conversation. When a significant pause presented itself, I took advantage. With Eric, our boys, Kenan and his family and Dee alongside, I swallowed the plum-like lump in my throat, sent a tranquil brainwave to my intestinal jitters, and dialed up Will. Thankfully he answered the bell, I broke the news to my parents with my uncle hanging on to my every word, and that part of my breast cancer journey was behind me. It is said that "life's problems wouldn't be called 'hurdles' if there wasn't a way to get over them." There were plenty more hurdles to face, but being forthright, honest, and composed was 'my way' of clearing this one. My parents were understandably curious, upset, shocked, and completely supportive. My uncle was noticeably angry. He resents and deplores breast cancer. He had a ringside seat to my aunt's battle. She never surrendered until breast cancer delivered the final blow. She was and always will be a champion of this insidious epidemic. I'll never forget 3 words he enforced..."Do the chemo". My aunt didn't and he believes if she had, the outcome may have been different. I brushed those words off at the time, but they wouldn't be the last time I'd hear them. Next stop, 24

18

hours later in Walpole MA. I had to tell my baby sister Julie...BREATHE.

That Monday, May 8, 2006 was possibly the longest Monday on record in my mind. Sure I tried to busy myself with work in the morning. I was the Child Care Supervisor at our gym. Afterschool activities, baseball, dinner and karate didn't prevent me from obsessive clock watching. Julie, Steve and my twin nieces were arriving at Logan International Airport, Boston around 9:30 p.m. Though it was late, I planned to drive to their house at 11:00 p.m. estimating their drive from Boston to Walpole. I didn't want to startle them, but I needed to tell my sister in person so I could assure her I was and would be o.k. My anxiety on the 20 minute ride from Mansfield to Walpole was palpable. It stemmed from an overwhelming need to protect her emotions. I was worried about her, and I hadn't told her anything yet. I called on my friend Will again. Will Power became one of my closest adversaries over the next few months. I arrived, parked, and knocked without ringing the doorbell. The twins were only 5 and after a long trip, I assumed they were sleeping. Jules answered and immediately knew some sort of trauma existed in our familiar world. Why else would I be there that late at night, right when they got home from a trip? Steve stood quietly while I embraced my baby sister on the couch and told her I had breast cancer. It took about 5 minutes for the wind to catch hold of her sails. I thought telling my parents and children were the hardest things I'd ever done. Telling Julie was equally as hard. Informing my baby sister that I had a life threatening disease was, quite possibly, one of the most emotionally taxing, gut wrenching things I've ever done. She wept with trepidation sensitively attempting to curb my feelings. Steve left the room. He was gone for about 15 minutes and in that time I conveyed to Julie my willingness to fight this bastard, my anger toward it, my hunger for information about it, my resolution to get our parents through it, and my promise that I'd win. Steve came back, gave me a bolstering hug, and then let my sister rest in his comforting shoulders. I heard her whisper, "What are we gonna do?" He answered without words. He simply crimped the tears from his eyes and continued to shelter her. I realized on my ride home why Steve reacted with such compassion. He had lost a brother in a motorcycle accident. He couldn't watch Julie endure the same heartache. He was good to have on my team too. In fact, Steve would quietly become one of my biggest supporters, in ways only he and I knew about, until now. I slept surprisingly well that night.

CHAPTER TWO

The next morning I worked, knowing I would share the news with my mother-in-law at lunch. Eric had the day off and invited her over. Before doing that, there was one more person I wanted to tell in person. Susie had become one of my closest friends. We met through my cousin, in 1993 and saw each other sporadically for several years after that. It wasn't until our sons started Little League that we became tight. We discovered that we grew up with very similar backgrounds, held our children to high standards and expectations, believed in the same core values, and appreciated each other implicitly. The most exciting connection, though, was our obsessive love for the Red Sox! She was the only woman I knew who could talk baseball with me for hours. We were up on all the stats, scoreboard, rosters, standings and latest news throughout the season. We knew every player's number, who they married or divorced, and even kept informed on the coaching staff and front office! We listened to sports radio any time we were driving and were avid sports column fans. It was incredible to share the Red Sox 2004 World Series Championship with Susie! I called her after work and asked if I could pop over for a few minutes. Luckily she was home and said 'yes'. When I got there she was outside on her front stoop. She greeted me with her blinding white smile and I acted as normally as I could. We went into her kitchen and Susie said,

"So, what's up?" I remember looking down so I wouldn't cry, and she said, "It's not cancer is it?" I looked at her beautiful face, put my hand on my heart, and said "m hm." I was in protective mode again. Susie had lost her best friend to breast cancer and I didn't want to be a blatant reminder. She then said, "Don't cry, don't cry" and I wiped my soon to be runny nose, brushed my pointer fingers across where eye liner would be drawn below my eyes, and we hugged. It didn't take me long to realize that Susie would become my personal suppository, up my ass on a consistent basis, in the best way possible! I then went home, joined Eric and Carol, my mother-in-law, for lunch in our kitchen, and gave Eric a little wink when I was ready to open the flood gates. Carol, a breast cancer survivor herself, has been through many ailments.

When she is told daunting news about a family member, the wind tends to switch direction on her and how she'll be affected. I couldn't let that happen. I needed her support and to be in MY corner. I couldn't have Eric worrying about her anxiety or sleeplessness, nor could I do that. Well, she pulled one out of her hat! Once hearing about what was in store for us, she continued to reassure me that I'd be 'fine', I'd beat this, and that she'd be there for us in whatever way she could...WHEW.

My news started making its way around town. The phone calls were constant. I realized I needed face time with one more person before she heard about me through the rumor mill. My neighbor Julie is a source of strength for so many in our community. She puts together food trains for families in need. I was one of her volunteer cooks. I knew she'd want to turn the tables and organize a food train for our family once she heard my diagnosis. I was right, and then some! Julie was a comforting listener, and made it less difficult for me to tell her. Then, almost immediately she put her conductor's hat on and went to work! By the end of that week she had organized a meal schedule to be provided by over 60 volunteers. We'd eventually received 3 meals a week for the course of my treatment! This brought us right up to Christmas time. It was an incredible gift and such a humbling part of my journey that I will never, ever, forget.

May 11, 2006 was the 'meeting of the minds'. This was the day we'd learn exactly what gateways were available to arrive at destination: freedom. Since learning of my diagnosis just a week earlier, a fire had ignited inside me. I was the same mom, wife, sister, friend, daughter that I always was, BUT, I had changed as a whole woman. I became obsessed with beating this monster. I wanted to start the engine and get moving. Eric and I met with each specialist individually that morning. They had convened before we arrived to conclude what my treatment plan would include, with the best statistical outcome. Each physician examined me individually and did a complete manual breast exam. FOUR times I got felt up in a matter of $\frac{1}{2}$ hour by FOUR different doctors! That hadn't happened since some innocent teenage exploration in middle school! Obviously this was important for their decisions and I was just trying to humor myself. After consulting with my surgeon, my oncologist, a radiation oncologist and a patient advocate we had our answers. Those 3 words my uncle had said, "Do the chemo", were chanting in my head. I asked the oncologist the success rates of my type of cancer, the location of it and the remission rate if chemo was tabled. Dr. Browne answered me in numbers and statistics and then she actually said, "Noreen, do the chemo". It was only the second time in knowing my husband that I saw him cry. He's not an outwardly emotional man. Seeing him tear up was a clear indication how deeply this was affecting him and how reality was uncomfortably setting in. Eric then said, "Noey, do the chemo". Decision made. So, the deal was that I would undergo a lumpectomy to remove the tumor on May 24th (what I now consider my survivor anniversary). While in surgery the surgeon would implant a port to receive chemotherapy through my veins and perform a sentinel node biopsy to determine if I had lymph node involvement. I would be given a few weeks to recover, and then begin 8 rounds of chemotherapy to be followed with 6 weeks of radiation then wrap it up with a prescription for 5 years of Tamoxifen, (which after $1\frac{1}{2}$ years switched to Arimidex). I'd cross the finish line around Christmas... LET'S GO.

I spent the days leading up to the surgery working at the gym, telling my boss and certain members I'd become friendly with about my cancer, scorekeeping my son Clay's baseball games, attending karate and lacrosse for the boys, and planning for the impending, inevitable changes about to come. The internet became my friend and enemy all at once. I was so curious about my particular breast cancer, risk of reoccurrence, chemo side effects, percentages etc. that I developed information overload. It was not good. It was bad. It was anxiety inducing (or extending in my case) to the point that Eric banned me from the computer! I also was feeling very nostalgic. My close friend Kerry from high school was a constant on my mind. We attended college together where people would always mistake us for sisters. We were in each other's weddings. She watched Zack when he was an infant while I worked. Then as the years went on our communication became sporadic. We always remembered to touch base on birthdays, anniversaries and Christmas but we didn't see each other much. I missed her. She could make me laugh more than anyone I ever knew, and still can. I refuse to get Botox because she's responsible for some of my laugh lines that I never want to lose! One is even named after her! I called Kerry the night before my surgery and broke the news. One in eight women was diagnosed with breast cancer in 2006. Kerry, knowing this statistic, said "thanks for taking the bullet for me". I appreciated her humor and knew it was her way of dealing. She also said "I'm so bad at this stuff but just know you can call me if you need anything". She remains one of my best girlfriends today. The morning of my surgery at Newton/Wellesley Hospital, I was strangely calm, for me. We pulled into the parking garage before 7:30 a.m. and I needed to call Cara in Pittsburgh to say a strong 'hi'. Cara feels helpless in these situations because of the miles between us and I wanted to reassure her I was at ease, eager to get this son of a bitch out of me, and move on to phase 2. She was understandably emotional, but we hung up with clear confidence and a promise I (or Eric) would speak to her after I got home. We entered the hospital to register and as I was filling out paperwork at the front desk, I remember feeling familiar sensory warmth behind me. I turned to find Julie, my sister, waiting there for us before she went to work. She said she just needed to see me and hug me good luck. That's when I lost it a bit. I was, in that moment, infinitely grateful for my family. I felt truly blessed that my sister would put me first on her busy calendar. I said my see you later to Jules and headed up with Eric to pre-op. From past experiences, this is where I usually develop annoying feathers in my chest and my palms get slimy. I didn't. I was on a mission...GET IT OUT!

They did. Port was implanted. Sentinel node was negative. THANK GOD. The sentinel node is considered the gatekeeper to the lymph nodes. If there was any evidence in that particular biopsy of extended lymph node involvement, my prognosis may have been completely different. It was time to recover and go home. I needed to follow up with my surgeon in a week, then begin chemo 6/19/2006. During that time I was encouraged to make a chemo 101 appointment at my infusion center. That was tons of fun. I learned all the 'could happens' of chemotherapy side effects and what's done to manage them. Of course I convinced myself that I'd get all of them, but then countered my own thinking and insisted that I'd blow all the odds. I'd do everything in my power to avoid the wretched byproducts of chemotherapy. It was another self-imposed belief that if I skated through with minimal treatment induced reactions, I'd be victorious over little bin. I just did what I could with what I had. I learned from my breast surgeon the pathology of my cancer at my post-surgery follow up. It was a .6 cm tumor, stage 1, invasive lobular carcinoma, grade 3. The size was small. The staging was early. The grade was bad. Grade 3 meant that my tumor had a high risk of metastasis. Tumors are graded based on how the surrounding cells and tissue appear under a microscope. My tumor was poorly differentiated which means abnormal

35

looking cells and lacking tissue structure. It would grow and spread fast. A wave roared through me. I understood in that moment that if I hadn't had the MRI, the tumor would've kept spreading, fast and undetected. Dr. Jill saved my life. I truly would've continued relying on annual mammograms, which never, ever would've shown my cancer. It hides in the lobules, behind the milk ducts. It's a mean fucking monster. Of course mammograms are vital for many types of breast cancer and I advocate, and will forever, how important they are. I just require an annual MRI along with an annual mammogram, as is now recommended for my sisters. They have the same family history I do and now have me as part of our history too. During this month of medical merry go round our family decided to attend the annual Relay for Life.

Our neighbor Jon is a cancer survivor who went through hell but kept on going. He was the keynote speaker that year. He and his wife formed the team Lifesavers. He kicked ass with his speech! I secretly hoped that someday I would be brave enough to deliver such a personal, powerful message. My news had gotten around town and it seemed like Mansfield in its entirety was on the track that night. There were many well-wishers, friends, colleagues and neighbors routing me on. I promised myself that I'd be on the 2007 committee come hell or high water. I wanted and needed to contribute to our town Relay as my small way of giving back.

CHAPTER THREE

After some minor discomfort post-surgery, I prepared myself for my 1st chemo treatment, as scheduled, 6/19/2006. I wanted to bring some levity to the party so I inscribed the words 'TRY ME' on my port with a sharpie! I took all of the anti-nausea meds that would help ward off the spins that the A/C (Adriamycin/Cytoxan) may cause. Eric and I left our house, nerves in check, and headed north to begin the next stop on my 'kick the CAN' out of CANcer quest. After signing in at the infusion center, paying the co-pay, and sitting in the waiting area, a nurse called my name. I remember my brain doing a mental dance where it couldn't find its footing. I wasn't nervous, just in a seemingly unbreakable haze. She led me to the pretreatment room where blood is drawn before every infusion, and the weeks in between. Since this was my inaugural takeoff into chemotherapy, my blood and all counts within were perfect to launch. DRIP, DRIP, DRIP...

Dr. Browne, my oncologist, met with us in her office before leading us to chemo camp. She estimated when my hair would begin to fall out, suggested wig outlets, reminded me of the mouth sores I may begin to incur and prescribed the appropriate rinse. She also informed us that because the white cell count dramatically drops as chemo attacks my cellular system, it'd be in my best medical interest to receive 4 injections of

Neulasta, a white cell builder. I'd have a choice. I could take the injection at home, within 24 hours of chemo OR I could take the injection at the infusion center within 24 hours of chemo. Well, of course I wanted Eric to give it to me at home. I didn't know how I'd be feeling and at least that small sense of security being home was a comfort. What Dr. Browne didn't impart was the financial burden that accompanied these injections if taken outside the medical facility...what? The 1st day of treatment wasn't horrible but it was emotionally daunting. I was doing ok until Katie, my beautiful nurse, injected the sludge through my port. No going back. I was now on my trek through this life altering odyssey. I remember feeling sad. I never told Eric because I didn't want him feeling bad for me. He had enough stress

to shoulder. It hit me right at the moment
the needle punctured my skin, POP. I could
get really sick from this shit ass garbage.
I could lose more weight than I should. My
body would not be the same, and it wasn't.
I would receive glares from onlookers. I
was a uniquely wrapped cancer patient with
all the trimmings, or eventually would be. I
quickly shifted mental gears and focused on
the outcome of being cancer free. Eric
went and got us a nice lunch and we spent
the rest of the session talking to the
nurses and other patients. I was exhausted
and somewhat loopy on the way home so we
called a friend to bring dinner over. The
next morning I remember thinking that I
COULD do this. I knew my hair would fall
out, most likely on our trip to Pittsburgh. I
opted for bandanas, baseball caps and big
earrings over a wig. I'd get the rest I

needed and I wouldn't let pride stand in my way. If I did that, cancer would get a leg up. I'd continue to LIVE my life, with acute caution regarding my health. I'd attend social events, the beach, and enjoy my family. One thing I stored in a small room in the back of my mind was that chemotherapy is cumulative. Each subsequent treatment attacks more and more cells, and the effects build up in one's body. I spent 4 hours on the phone the Friday after my chemo initiation with my insurance company, a patient advocate, and a pharmacist fighting against the $14,000.00 Neulasta would set our family back simply because I chose, as a cancer patient, to receive it at home. It turns out that it's covered, except for the office copay, if chosen to receive it at the infusion center. So, after 4 hours of tears, arguments, rage, and demanding reasonable explanation, I accomplished my 1st of several battles with insurance. I'd be charged only what I would've been if I'd gone to Wellesley, $35.00 per shot. That's a $13,860.00 difference! I learned a hard fought lesson that afternoon. I had to stand in the batter's box and swing for the fences myself. I felt ok, with a little fatigue after week one at camp. It was estimated that my hair would fall out during the 1st week of July. We would be in Pittsburgh celebrating the 4th of July with Cara, Bill, Bryer and Jarrett. Bryer was 15. I had all these visions of clumps of my hair around their house. I was freaking out about it. I was concerned Bryer would freak out too. Teenagers ride enough emotional rollercoasters. I didn't need to take her on mine too. It takes about 10 hours to drive to Pittsburgh from Mansfield. Prior to leaving I decided to ask a friend if she'd come over and cut my hair short. I thought this would make the transition from long hair to baby bald an easier pill to swallow...GULP.

We set out on 7/2/2006 to drive to Cara's. About half ways into the trip my head felt like a swarm of fleas had infested it. It also felt a strange sense of coolness similar to a freshly shaven leg. I kept this to myself, but Eric couldn't help but notice my incessant scratching. The boys were in the back seat and were thankfully oblivious. This was the red alert of my bald invasion. I called it that because I was defenseless to this attack. Going bald came with the territory and I wasn't armed with any retaliatory means except the choices I made on how to wear it. When we arrived at my sister's she greeted us at the front door. She gushed over my short haircut and I accepted the praise without telling her I'd be buzzing it off, myself, the next morning. We enjoyed a nice dinner. Bill's cousins were visiting at the same time but they stayed at Bill's dads down the street. I'm not one who usually is selfish, but I didn't want to share Cara on this trip. I wanted Bill's cousins to either go home to the west part of the country or at the very least, leave us alone. They didn't. I vented my frustration to Eric, who is less selfish than me, and surprisingly he felt the same way! We decided to get over it and enjoy our time with our family. I asked Bill if he had a buzzer before I went to bed. He kindly left it on the bathroom counter I was sharing with Bryer. I woke up before everyone the next morning and buzzed my head. When my friend cut my hair I felt a little nervous but I knew it was only hair. It would grow back. I didn't want the cancer to. When I buzzed my own head I felt empowered. I was taking control of this pesky interloper. I was giving the finger to cancer. I spent less than a minute shedding some tears then actually smiled at my new whiffled self in the mirror. Then I loudly whispered "Fuck you little bin". That was the nickname I gave my tumor because it had infiltrated my breast. It was a terrorist. We removed it on May 24th but its siege on my body was continual. I got some gym clothes on, went in the family room and practiced yoga. I didn't put a bandana or baseball cap on because my boys had to see me as me. They needed to get accustomed to my look because my hair wouldn't begin growing back until after chemo. I still wasn't even bald yet! That would come later when we got home. One by one everybody awoke. Eric saw me first and said I was lucky I had a 'good head'. I know he meant it. I also know that people, especially those closest to you, don't know the right thing to say. Well guess what, there is NO right thing to say. I expected my family to shower me with compliments and they exceeded what I anticipated. This outpouring of support and love was, on that day, my breakfast of fortitude. I drank their moxie...POWER ON.

We decided to go to a local Japanese Hibachi restaurant that night for dinner without Bill's cousins. I wore a black shirt, jeans and a silk scarf tied to the side of my

head. On a quick trip to the ladies room
with Cara she sweetly tried to comfort me.
She said "This look is something you'd wear
anytime". I balked at her comment while
looking in the mirror. I swear mine was the
look Cher was channeling while writing
'Gypsies, Tramps and Thieves'! That's what
was screaming back at me from the mirror.
Gypsy! I snidely snapped at Cara saying
"I'd never wear anything like this". I saw
Little Niagara begin to flow from her
bounteous eyes so we both agreed I was
right and went on to enjoy a fun night out
with our family. The next day Bill and Cara
had arranged for all of us to attend an
annual 4th of July party. Well, Mother
Nature had other things in mind beside
fireworks including a buffet of rain with all
the fixings! We were served king size
helpings of wind, thunder, lightning, and

enough rain to saturate the Mojave Dessert. Ms. Nature may have dampened our plans, but she illuminated our spirit. We spent the entire day eating, playing board games, and laughing. It was a perfect way to end our short stay in Pittsburgh. We left early the next morning not knowing when we'd see the Blumes again. I knew however, with every fiber of my being if I needed Cara to come to me she would. What neither one of us anticipated was when I would see her in August I'd truly look like a cancer patient. By then my eyebrows and lashes would've fallen out and I'd be cue ball bald and 9 pounds less. The ride home was uneventful. It took an entire day which gifted me a lot of time to think. I submerged myself into imagery pools of new looks I could create. Would I wear more makeup? Would I get a rainbow of bandanas? Would I draw on eyebrows and glue on eyelashes? Would I shield my scar? Would I whiten my teeth? Some of my answers were automatic NO's (like the teeth whitening) because of the chemo. A NO also answered shielding my scar. This was my survival wound from my lifesaving battle. I'd wear it proudly and openly. Others were automatic why Nots. Why not try false eyelashes? Why not pencil in some eyebrows? And why not darken my lip gloss? I'll tell you why not. None of those things were the essence of me. I had gotten my period the morning we left Cara's on July 5th, 2006. This would be the last cycle I'd ever endure. I was 44. I was content with my boys and we were done having children, especially after the miscarriage I had suffered 7 months prior to my cancer diagnosis. Still, why was this chemical cocktail allowed to induce such a nauseating muliebral hangover? My maternal fate was in its hands and I didn't like it. An early menopause is a common response to chemo. I was resentful but soon realized that not having a monthly period wasn't so bad. What were bad were the night sweats, hot flashes, mood swings and vaginal drought my body would incur. We arrived home, road weary. It was summer so it wasn't a school night. I went to bed soon after we got home. I'd get up early to shave my head...RAZOR PLEASE!

CHAPTER FOUR

The next morning I woke up a different woman. I thought buzzing my head in Pittsburgh was a power trip. I actually couldn't wait to shave it now! I used a disposable razor, doused my head with shaving cream, asked Will Power to stand beside me with Eric, and G.I Janed myself! It took about 2 minutes. It's funny. I remember my cousin losing her hair in the late 90's during her treatment. She never wore a wig. I actually thought, back then, that if I ever had to make that arduous decision in my life that I'd forgo the wig too. Foreshadowing is a strange occurrence. Here I was, in 2006, bald. That same cousin brought me over a bag of her scarves and every bandana on the color wheel. From that day on I'd be seen with a bandana and big earrings or a bandana and a baseball cap or occasionally a silk scarf. My skin on my head was thankfully smooth. That was a Wednesday morning. Three days later we were expected at a friend's house for a backyard cookout. We knew most of the guest list, a bevy of beautiful women and men from our town and family/friends of our hosts. I spent a good portion of the days leading up to the party selecting the right outfit. It was all about the headwear! I chose my scarf then paired the rest. It would be our 1st social appearance since my inaugural treatment but I felt an innate craving for normalcy. I understood there would be curiosity and I'd receive a bit more attention. It was all good. I just didn't want to be THE

CANCER elephant in the room. The night arrived. I tied my scarf in a braid to the left side and wore especially long earrings. My eyelashes and eyebrows still remained so I brushed a few extra coats of mascara on, painted on some bronzer and drenched my lips in a cinnamon shaded high sheened gloss. I felt slightly self-conscious getting ready. The extra makeup strangely boosted my confidence. Usually I'd feel the opposite with that much shit on my face but I needed some semblance of attraction. Physically I felt fine. No side effects were creeping up on me, baldness withstanding! It was a gorgeous summer evening. I indulged in nice conversations with townsfolk and friends. One of my friends said to me "You're wearing much more makeup than usual". I simply responded that I was more comfortable with a little extra. Secretly I was embarrassed and horrified. The comment was made in front of a group of local women who know me to be fairly natural. Suddenly I felt like a circus freak. I felt anxiety symptoms start to run amuck in my body. Normally I'd have a cocktail to relax but I wasn't drinking, at all, during treatment. I made an excuse (having to pee) to escape my conundrum and found other friends inside. Eric met me at the party late because he had to work. He always worked Saturdays. In fact, since we were dating, one of us has always worked the weekends. We, as a couple, have never had weekends off. When he finally arrived at the party my nerves settled. I dismissed the earlier comment about my extra makeup and enjoyed the rest of the night. There weren't too many occasions after that where I needed to don more cosmetics than I'd normally use.

My eyebrows and lashes disappeared before my 2nd treatment, along with my pubes. Now I looked sick. I'm what many call money in the bank for a dermatologist because of my innately fair skin! I'm Casper white with hazel eyes. I NEED mascara to bring them out! This bothered me more than losing my hair. I was reconsidering the false eyelashes that I balked at before. Cheryl, Susie's twin sister came over with her bead making kits and false eyelashes. Susie came too. We spent an afternoon crafting earrings which Che was kind enough to let us keep. Troy got in on the fun when he got home. He and Che created a mock shop of earrings for me to patronize. I selected a couple of pairs (that I knew Troy handmade). Then it was time for Eyelash Gluing Academy. Che was clearly an expert on it and I clearly was not! She generously left some eyelashes and glue with my promise to her that I'd continue to try. Chemo #2 was in a few days. Should I surprise all the nurses and come adorned for camp, lashes and all? One of my nurses, Katie, was breathtakingly beautiful with pools of blue where her eyeballs should be. Her skin was flawless. Her smile illuminated the room. And, to pour fresh squeezed lemon juice in that cut, she was genuinely nice too. One would think I'd be self-conscious around such a vision when I certainly didn't look my best! She had the opposite effect. She inspired me to bake little treats on each infusion day for all the nurses, doctors, and aides. It made me feel good to help them

57

feel appreciated. After all, they are in the business of saving lives and fostering hope. It was the least I could do to extend a sweet offering every 3 weeks. Susie would chauffer me to my 2nd treatment. I made chocolate chip cheesecake brownies for the staff. I had my Livestrong binder, lunch bag, book and other necessities prepared to go. I wore my new pink Red Sox baseball cap complete with the breast cancer ribbon the Rae family had gifted me. Steve had also sent me a new CoCo Crisp t-shirt because I'd mentioned how I loved his name. The Red Sox had acquired Crisp that season with high hopes...hmph. I left the eyelashes and makeup at home...LET'S GO!

Mouth sores? Check. Did I have minor weight loss? Check. Salient senses? Check. (It was akin to pregnancy when the slightest whiff of pizza, pork, or Chinese food would initiate a hangover effect). This was the point in my treatment when 'Cancer Magazine' could've called on me to be their cover girl. I was approached by strangers telling me 'you're not alone' or 'we're all here to get you through it' or 'my wife/sister/mom/grandmother etc. is a survivor'. I couldn't believe my personal war was so far out on the front lines. I felt naked, except for my bandana. It was the middle of July so the boys' sports had wrapped up. Eric's work schedule was (and still is) a retail one. He didn't get home until 7:00 pm most days and worked every other Sunday. I leaned on close friends (Susie/Lynn), neighbors and family more than ever. The cumulative effect of chemo was beginning to show its ugly face so I tried to shield it by staying as mentally and

physically strong that I could. Every
morning, without fail, I would go On
Demand and find a yoga routine, usually
instructed by Rodney Yee. Aside from
Ellen Degeneres, he became my TV savior.
I watched Ellen religiously, from her show's
premiere in 2003 with Jennifer Aniston
until today. Actually, I've been a front
runner for her #1 fan since seeing her
LIVE in Boston. She was in town for the
Here and Now tour. Let's just say I
should've remembered Depends! I've really
followed her career since she was on
Johnny Carson and Open House, a sitcom
about real estate. Ellen was a force of
nature for me during treatment. The
laughter she invoked and the magnanimous
humanity she displayed was medicinal
nirvana for me! I watched the repeats all
summer and couldn't wait for the

September premiere! I think it was from Central Park in 2006, city to the dreaded New York Yankees but because it was Ellen, I forgave her! She was and is a goddess to me. Her mom Betty is a breast cancer survivor so I do feel an intrinsic connection to her. It sounds cheesy but I do have a bucket list and meeting Ellen is top priority on it, (as is kickin' back with Lenny Kravitz but for different reasons)! My lust for Lenny is no secret to Eric. We've agreed that he's my hall pass and Eric's is J. Lo! Who knows, maybe someday the 5 of us will cross paths together. Or, maybe not, but a girl can dream! Even if I only could manage 10 or 15 minutes of yoga, I did it. I did it for strength. I did it for release. I did it for power. I did it because I did it. I quickly developed an addiction to yoga and used it as part of my defense. It truly helped me fight breast cancer and became a bastion of reinforcement. I took a class called Centergy every Sunday morning at 9:00. My cousin (the breast cancer survivor) met me at the gym and we 'centergized' together. The first few classes were complimentary then I would have to sign a membership or pay as I go. My cousin realized that I couldn't afford either option, but appreciated that I needed this class. She secretly spoke with the manager and he gifted me an unlimited class membership for the remainder of my treatment. One of the many ways I witnessed people getting out of their own way and paying it forward. I certainly accepted his generous offer and continued to take Centergy, every Sunday, without fail. I even went when I was in a multi week river of diarrhea! I told Dr. Browne and

Katie, who Susie echoed my adoration for, about my mouth sores and the runs. Neither of them reacted with any sort of fervor. I guess this was just par for the course. Susie and I spent a nice afternoon in camp together. We read magazines, gossiped, swooned over Katie's beauty and chatted up a few of the other patients. If it weren't for the Drano being pumped through my veins, I would've called this a great 'girl's day out'! Upon leaving I was prescribed a special rinse for the mouth cankers, Mylanta, Imodium and a bevy of 'regulators' that ultimately didn't work. One of the nurses eventually said to me 'Nor look, I know that if I eat ice cream I'm going to have fierce cramps. I get a double scoop if I feel like it and deal with the cramps because it's worth it'. I believed her, followed her advice because I needed

to eat and eventually was back to normal
shits! Boy did that first no wiper feel
sweet! The rinse for the mouth sores did
the trick, very quickly so by my 3rd
treatment I was eating a somewhat normal
diet and my white and red blood cell counts
were within allowable range...IN YOUR
FACE!

CHAPTER FIVE

Our family life hadn't changed much in between the 2nd and 3rd treatments. Zack celebrated his 16th birthday. His favorite color has always been orange so I made him an orange cake. Throughout the years I've always baked the boys' birthday cakes and themed each one. They've noshed on Blue's Clues, Batman, Thomas the Train, Buzz Lightyear, Hogwarts, Big Bird, and the list goes on. Now 16, I figured Zack wouldn't want a childish cake, but I wanted my confectionary love in the batter regardless! He appreciated my efforts and I was grateful to surreptitiously coddle him on his birthday. My blood count and wellness visits were on par to this point. I didn't require Procrit (a red cell booster) and my white counts were perfect due to the golden Neulasta . I still shutter thinking about the insane cost to unknowing patients of that damned shot. It definitely aided in my tolerance of the chemo BUT it also could've set us back over $14,000.00, unbelievable. It was late July and the weather was hot! Neulasta, like chemo, is cumulative. It amps the white blood cells which means the 'medicine' seeps into the bones. I remember being chilled to my core one morning when the outside thermometer read 82 degrees. I was under all my bed coverings and an extra fleece blanket, shivering. The boys were home but I didn't want to worry them so I stayed in my room and relayed that I was especially tired that day. I called the infusion center and spoke with one of my nurses. She explained that this was a side effect of the Neulasta and to do what I could to get warm. It goes marrow deep, she conveyed, but the chills wouldn't last so try to motor through. I tried. I got out of bed, literally trembling. I decided my yoga may help so I went On Demand, found Rodney Yee, turned up the thermometer in our bedroom and practiced 20 minutes of yoga in my sweatshirt and leggings. I felt better. Not 100%, but better. Our above ground pool was a saving grace that summer. On the days my body felt quasi normal, I'd edge myself into the water ever so gingerly. It was such a relief on the opposite of Neulasta chill day. There were days that I couldn't bear the heat and humidity so the pool was just what the doctor ordered, literally! Lynn accompanied me to week 3 of chemo camp. By now I felt like a counselor in training. I knew the drill up down and sideways and found myself engaging in other patient's personal situations. I gave Lynn the rundown on the 40 minute drive there so she wouldn't be blindsided. If you've never been a camper at this non-exclusive camp, the probability to be sucker-punched is high. Lynn is a single mom of 3 and tends to waste no time or energy confronting things head on. She was a leader on my team. She also melts like butter in the sun when affected by sensitive issues close to her heart. We had to keep her solid because she was a vital link in my chain of strength. I continued to bring treats to the nurses, which gave me a psychological boost, and flapped my social butterfly wings with the other patients. Lynn was/is a fiercely loyal employee. She brought her laptop with her to complete some work, but ended up foregoing that and engaging in whatever I wanted to do. We watched TV, ate lunch, watched a movie on her laptop, and conversed with the other campers. I know how dedicated Lynn is to her work and how diligent she is about it. She sacrificed a day of work for me which plucked at the strings in my heart. I talked to she and Susie everyday which to me, was like taking multi vitamins. They supplied me with all the necessary supplements! The next few weeks would prove to be my most challenging yet. We were now in August and humidity had set in. My red cells were beginning to decline and I'd have to forgo this one part of my chemo competition and succumb to an injection of Procrit. I wanted to get through my entire treatment without it so I could have bragging rights. Then I did a full 360 and thought, 'who the hell cares'? The Procrit boosted my red blood cells, which in turn, helped me endure the remainder of this Drano diet. My body felt like a pin cushion by now so what was one more shot every 3 weeks? August 21st would be my 4th and final serving of A/C chemo. The Blumenscheins visited from Pittsburgh in between my 3rd and 4th treatments. I looked sick to them. The rest of my family had VIP seats to my transition from 44 year old decent looking, fit and toned, long haired blonde Noah to bald, eyelash-less, eyebrow-less, thin, pale, sullen cancer patient. Cara, Bill and the kids had seen me only a month earlier but the change in my appearance hit them like a Red Sox Pedro Martinez fastball to the face. We still had a long way to go. PLAY BALL!

It must've been the hottest, most humid day of 2006. My girlfriends from high school were coming for a visit. Unfortunately the rest of my family was heading to Kenan's for a pool day with the Blumenscheins and Uncle Charlie and Carol. Eric strongly encouraged me to cancel on my friends but I hadn't seen them since long before I'd gotten sick and was relishing the thought of laughing with them. Plus, I didn't want to be subjected to the extreme weather amongst my nieces, nephew and parents. I knew I'd melt like the Wicked Witch and truly wanted to stay home. I knew I'd see Cara the next day, when it was forecasted to be tolerable. Well, my friends rescheduled. Learning this Eric was relentless. He didn't want to leave me alone at home. He simply didn't understand or could fathom the discomfort

I guaranteed I'd feel. I caved. I left the soothing central air conditioning and headed to Marshfield to bake. It wasn't anybody's fault. Kenan and Shelby have a refreshing pool that I was free to jump in but the roundabouts of motion sickness from the car, the dead air and the heat had already begun to circle. This sucked the royal big one. Everybody enjoyed pool games, good eats, and fun while I curled up like a snail on my brother's couch. My head spun while my body decorated itself with beads of sweat. The sounds of my family's laughter were another reminder of how this fucking disease was robbing me of what is most precious, time. I remember nimbly making my way to the back deck to signal to Eric I needed to go home. This, of course, sounded the alarms! My sister, Bill, Kenan, Shelby, Eric and my parents stopped what they were doing to come to my 'aid'. I just wanted to go home. Again, I didn't want to feel like the 'cancer' elephant in the room. My young niece, Shealyn, got me an ice pack. My mom wrapped her loving arms around me and my dad did what he does best, understood my need for space. I ached for my parents at this moment. You never want to feel helpless when your child is in distress. What was a few minutes seemed like hours that they all rallied around me, stared, and continued to ask if I was ok. My dad stood by me but left me alone. Truth be told, I just needed to get the hell out of there. Kenan politely backed everyone off. I wore the ice pack like an Easter bonnet and began to cool down. Another weight on my shoulder was that my uncle and his wife remained in the back yard during all of this. I knew why. I was channeling my auntie Marguerite right in front of him and he just couldn't bear it. I called him the next day to apologize. Even that was awkward. I was trying to convey that I felt bad about not being my normally effusive self. Charlie was receptive to my regrets, but reserved in his response. We ended the conversation by me promising our next visit would be better. He and Carol share time between the east and west coasts so I didn't know when I'd see them again, but I was confident I'd be much better. The next visit to the infusion center was filled with everything negative. I couldn't have been happier! A few weeks into my treatment it was recommended I undergo genetics testing for BRCA1 and BRCA2 gene mutations that if positive, could ultimately affect my sisters, mom, female cousins, nieces and me. I agreed to the testing after Dr. Browne cited the statistics and assured me that if I were her sister, she'd insist she do it. It was a simple blood test, but, again was insurance prohibitive and another battle I had to wage. Plus, if I did have a positive mutation of these specific genes, my ovaries, breasts, uterus and overall reproductive system would be in potential jeopardy. Family history was again, a factor. Some women opt to forgo these genetics tests if no family history is presented or for any number of personal reasons. It came down to an individual, carefully scrutinized choice for me. I received negative results and was able to get the entire $3,000.00 test covered. Battle won! Katie and Dr. Browne prepped me for the next type of chemo cocktail they'd be serving for 'happy hour', Taxol. I was done with A/C treatments and officially half way through my summer of savage! Taxol would bring a new gift bag of side effects to the party but I was ready to change things up. It was not nausea inducing didn't invite mouth sores or promote fatigue. It did infiltrate bones, joints and muscles. I had the next three weeks to prepare for the Taxol, with blood work visits in between. I drove myself to these in between visits, but one day I wished I had company. A vicious hemorrhoid had bubbled up on my butt that was a result of the diarrhea I had endured. I presumed it would deflate as the weeks passed, but it did the opposite. What was supposed to be a routine blood work and check in visit with Dr. Browne landed me on a surgeon's table having a thumbrosed vessel removed from the hemorrhoid. Dr.

Browne examined the area and said "that's impressive" then sent me immediately to a surgeon Dr. Jill recommended. I didn't know this surgeon. I was alone. And I was in a precarious position to say the least! It makes me smile thinking back on it now, but on that day, I was not laughing. I didn't even call Eric until the whole ordeal was over and I got home. Thank God for my meal delivery angels that night! I was exhausted, frustrated, and had a very sore asshole! Just another hurdle to get over in this journey, and I cleared it. There were now 2 more weeks until my Taxol infusion which my parents had offered to accompany me to. I was grateful they were taking me, but uneasy about what their reaction may be. I was 44 but I was still their little girl. How could they watch me take injections, IV, pills, among the other patients for over 4 hours? I gave them several opportunities to cancel, but they didn't. Taxol Tuesday arrived. My mom and dad got to my house early. We went over the check list and headed north for a day that they, nor I, could ever have imagined. HUSH LITTLE BABY...

CHAPTER SIX

We arrived to the NEHO center. I signed
in at the desk, paid my $35 copay, and fell
into a flop sweat. The gentleman in front
of me had just completed his Taxol infusion
and was experiencing frightening
repercussions. His daughter and wife were
by his side. I asked Wendy, a nurse I'd
become comfortable with, if this would
happen to me. She reassured me it wouldn't
and that every patient's situation is unique.
I don't remember even hearing her. When
I experience anxiety I become an annoying
chatterbox with nonstop questions. I
wanted to cancel. I wanted to be done. I
wanted to wake up from this fucking
nightmare. My mom, who was a home health

aide and former gymnastics and dance coach reeled me back in. She, herself, dealt with severe bouts of anxiety and understood me. I could not and would not shut the hell up. I'd done my research on Taxol and the potential side effects. I anticipated the extra IV's of meds I needed prior to the actual Taxol infusion. There is a high probability of an allergic reaction to this septic shit, which is what I believe the man in the waiting room endured. I knew, personally, patients who had allergic reactions. It's fucking scary, Mom and Dad convinced me to get my prerequisite blood work done, have some water and talk to Katie. Katie was ultimately the one who convinced me to pregame with Ativan and anti-allergens to feel more comfortable about the Taxol. I did fine, with the exception of the

nonsensical state I was drug induced into.
I was in Ativan haze for the remainder of
the afternoon. Some people pay good coin
for this shit. I'm so sensitive to medication
that any kind of 'good' high is wasted on me.
I just get wasted! Mom and Dad did fine.
They did more than fine. See, they invoked
some sort of super power that day to
withstand what they witnessed. They were
comfortably accustomed to my appearance
but in the confines of an infusion center
your appearance mimics those around you.
Sick, struggling, stricken, battling warriors
and I was one of the troops. There I was,
their tow haired baby girl fighting a life
threatening disease. This IS the disease
that Mom watched her sister Marguerite
battle, 11 years prior. A disease, had it not
been for my breast MRI ordered by Dr.
Jill, would've quite possibly taken my life. A

disease I vehemently despise. My dad is a realist. He deals with issues as they arise and doesn't sweat the small stuff. My mom is the polar opposite. She worries about others. She is a fortress of angst and 'frets' the small stuff. I honestly thought I'd have to spend the day easing her distress but she spun the wheels. My parents were grand marshals in the parade of calm that day. I merely marched in line, on my little cancer float, and followed in step behind them. My dad read most of the day and left for a bit to bring back lunch. My mom busied herself talking to the other patients and their caregivers, Katie and any nurse who would engage her. All of them did! She watched a few shows and enjoyed non cancer related conversation with me. I recall a distinct feeling of relief and pride to have them with me. I was a mom of three sons but THAT day I was their oldest child of four, feeling like I was twelve being taken to the doctor by my parents. We celebrated my introduction to Taxol with a nap for me on the ride home! I fought sleep the entire day, much to Katie's frustration, and was overcome with exhaustion and Ativan withdrawal. It took less than an hour to get to Mansfield. Eric wasn't home from work yet but my parents wanted to head home instead of visiting. They were beat too. The next few weeks were filled with flag football for Troy and karate. The boys were back in school. Clay was reffing flag football and Zack was busy driving anywhere he could with his new learner's permit. The fact that my knees felt like David Ortiz, (or Big Papi to Red Sox nation) were taking batting practice on them didn't prevent me from attending all the boys' activities. I simply would NOT let this son of a bitch win. It was during this time, while sitting in a camp chair at Troy's flag football games and practices that I began to pen some thoughts about my journey with breast cancer. I will tell you how my words came to benefit breast cancer awareness later in my story. Let's just say that what you put out there truly does circle back around so why wouldn't you put out positivity? Karma is a boomerang so project wisely. Taxol had introduced itself to my joints in a forceful way, which I found quite rude, but ignored its obnoxious mannerisms and motored through. If not, cancer wins...NOT.

CHAPTER SEVEN

It was now the middle of October. I'd
endured 3 rounds of Taxol and weeks of
potty mouth inducing joint pain. Jules and I
set up a lunch date at a pub in between our
houses. I was so excited to spend some
time with her and forget about my cancer
treatment for an hour or two. We met in
the parking lot, hugged, and went in for an
anticipated nice lunch. We chatted for a
bit, and then ordered. Everything seemed
completely normal until I felt like I was
behind the safety bar of a tilt-a-whirl. The
food came and I tried to play it like things
were like any other lunch we had enjoyed
together, except they weren't. The spins
were increasing (without the induction of

alcohol), but shamefully, I didn't want to bother Julie with this. I tried my best to steady myself. I went to the ladies room to splash some water on my face. That didn't help. I came back to the table and took a bite of food. I gulped my water with lemon...nothing. I had to confess to her that I was in a whirlwind of apparent vertigo and in need of her help. This reeked of weakness to me but fortunately I was in the company of my sister and I was not sitting in judgment. According to her, I ruled no matter what. She was able to cool me off and was angelically patient. I finally regained my inner balance but we decided it'd be best if we got some 'to go' boxes and call it a day. I was so sad. I really wanted this to be special time with my baby sister and, once again, cancer disrupted my life. I felt like I had 'swass' because of all the wetness caused by my surf worthy tears driving home. It was a mixed batter of anger and despondence that cancer whisked up. It has no right to do that because its victims are sitting ducks. Cancer is a sneaky, painful, contemptible, sly coward. It hides and grows until it's discovered in one way or another. It doesn't show its ugly face unless it is found, or it has surfaced, or it has grown and spread too fast and too far, undetected. Did I mention how much I HATE and DEPLORE this disease? At my next appointment with Dr. Browne I explained to her what had happened at lunch, several days prior. Eric was with me, thank God because Dr. Browne stated it could be a Taxol related cardiac issue. Cardiac? Now my heart was in jeopardy? Dr. Browne left the room for a few minutes and I went into a complete frenzy. This was to be my last Taxol infusion day and instead I was presented with the possibility of my heart being compromised by this fucker. I'd had it. I told Eric I was done. I told Dr. Browne when she returned I was done. I threw the pillow from the exam table across her office and began to hyperventilate. She settled my Oscar worthy performance by referring me to the chief of cardiology at Newton Wellesley Hospital, immediately. She wanted this doctor to research the effects of Taxol to the heart, if given 3 of 4 treatments. Would my risk of reoccurrence increase? Would there be any significant altered risk? What were the statistics proving his confirmations? We left the infusion center and went directly to the hospital. I was seen immediately by a male nurse who was beyond awesome! He was funny, compassionate, sensitive, and perceptive to my amped anxiety. I was running on about 10,000 volts! He administered all the protocoled tests before I met with the top dog. I was hoping against hope this well respected, reputable cardiologist would have the news I wanted to hear, that my dance with chemo had taken its final turn on the floor. I wanted to hear that there were no cases that proved one more treatment of Taxol would benefit me or increase my risk of the bastard holding fort in my body again. Eric and I waited in his oversized 'room with a view' office for about 15 minutes. We didn't mind. It gave us time to breathe out and discuss our decisions pending what the doctor's research uncovered. We both agreed that if the stakes weren't raised by foregoing the 8th treatment then I would stop chemo. That's exactly what happened. He had to confer with Dr. Browne of course and was kind enough to put her on speaker phone so we could be part of the conversation. Dr. Browne was completely comfortable with his findings and recommendation that I stop chemo, with one exception. I had to wear a heart monitor for 30 days as a cautionary measure that nothing else was aggravating the ticker. Deal. The dizziness seemed to vanish, the monitor showed no abnormalities, and I was done with pumping liquid crap through my veins. I appreciate and am grateful for the available medicine that kept cancer at bay and temporarily killed my cellular system. I'm so angry that there is a global epidemic causing so many to suffer through these types of treatments. I'm a huge fan of alternative treatment, holistic medicine, clean green eating and exercise. Unfortunately, sometimes it just isn't enough and we have to follow 'doctor's orders' for the best possible outcome. The monitor came off in a month. Dr. Partridge removed the port as an outpatient surgery and my next chapter was about to begin, radiation therapy.

CHAPTER EIGHT

We are huge Halloween lovers in the Taranto household. Our home became one of the highly anticipated houses for trick or treaters in our neighborhood and surrounding towns as well. Parents would drop carloads of kids off in our block with highlights being our house and a few of our neighbors who also pulled out all the stops. Over the years we created themes like Haunted Forest, Grandma's Hotel Room, Star Wars, Creepy Diner, Swampland, Spiderweb, Curse of the Red Sox and more. Once we even had a bouncy house in the front yard which I hid in dressed like an escaped prisoner! I didn't want this year to be any different. Troy had turned 9 on

August 18th. He was still very much into Halloween and enjoyed the attention he received on the school bus the day after. He wanted to be a big part of planning this year's idea so he and I devised a sneaky plot to trick all of our neighbors! The family decided on American Idol as our theme. About 2 weeks before Halloween Troy and I went around with a video camera claiming he was doing a project for school and needed our friends' help. No we didn't! We actually got them to sing on camera, with not one of them questioning his idea. Then, on Halloween Zack, Eric and Clay rigged up TV's, cables, sound system and cameras to play back what Troy had captured on tape. Eric was 'Randy'. Zack was 'Simon' and I was 'Paula'. Zack's friend Ben was Ryan Seacrest, outside with a microphone! The trick or treaters would have to 'audition' their costumes for us to get their candy. It was a blast and great for me because I started radiation therapy the next day and all the hullaballoo distracted me from my anxiety. Plus, I felt kind of sexy in my Paula wig, slathered on makeup and funky dress! The neighbors got a kick out of seeing themselves on TV (with one exception of a mom who was embarrassed). She got over it! After we all changed, sifted through all the candy Troy and Clay collected and cleaned up it was time for bed. I was restless because I'd wake up and it'd be radiation day. One comforting thought was that I had already had my initial consultation with my radiation oncologist, Dr. Tom and I absolutely adored him. Julie had come with me for my first appointment at Rhode Island Hospital a couple of weeks after I stopped chemo.

We met Nurse Nancy who reviewed the side effects of this intensity-modulated radiation therapy (IMRT) and how to avoid them. She gave me extra strength Aquaphor, suggested bras, and since my job was in the child center of a gym she thought I'd ride this wave more successfully if I refrained from returning to work until I coasted into shore. I objected to this. I thought it'd be good for me to get back on the horse but both Nurse Nancy and Jules convinced me to hold off until this final leg was over. After that appointment, I needed to return to be tattooed in the precise area the beams would target. Susie took me to this appointment when we met Dr. Tom. He treated me like we were meeting at a cookout. The first thing I noticed was his bow tie! I would never come to see him without one. He introduced himself as Tom, asked Susie and I to sit down, shook both of our hands and secured eye contact with me which he never veered from. He was sympathetic to my nerves and such a calming presence in the sterile room we were conferring in.   I was about to be placed on yet another machine to determine where to inject the pen point sized tattoo on my right breast. They had to get this right. I knew it. The techs knew it. Susie knew it and Dr. Tom certainly knew it.   I began to tear up a bit and Dr. Tom actually wiped my tears, covered my hand with his and promised me this procedure would be painless and congratulated me for how much I'd already overcome. Aside from Dr. Jill, I'd never met a physician like him. I honestly felt like I was in the company of an angel. And the cherry on the sundae was that he was a HUGE Red Sox fan! Again, I could've done the radiation anywhere. Dr. Browne recommended Dr. Tom and I completely trusted her. She had gotten me the best of the best to this point. I was able to get through the tattoo unscathed and fell into Susie's warm welcoming arms when I hopped off the cold table. She couldn't contain her adulation for Dr. Tom and I agreed with her wholeheartedly. We talked about him most of the way back to Mansfield. I honestly don't think I would've done as well as I did through this journey of SUCK if Susie wasn't riding shotgun the entire way. She exemplified the genuine meaning of 'friend', was at my beck and call, checked in every single day without fail, and thankfully was one of my team leaders. I will never forget her compassion or her way of stepping in for my family and me. I love her. I love the way Syd and Claire reared her, Che and Rich, and though she was better situated than me economically, it didn't matter to her or me. We were both cut from non-expensive but premium quality cloth. The next couple of weeks were busy with Halloween planning, school projects and activities and enjoying life. Radiation would begin November 1st and finish December 13, Susie's birthday! The October Halloween moon slowly gave way to the November sunrise and, though it was chilly out I could feel the heat rising. Radiation had arrived...one, two, three ZAP!

The half hour drive to Rhode Island Hospital 5 days a week for 7 weeks never really got to me. There's a reason for that. I had company almost every single time. Susie drove me along with my cousin, my sister, Lynn, my friend Wendy, Eric, my neighbor, and other volunteers. Some days I would take myself which was fine. I never truly experienced the fatigue associated with radiation therapy. I got a little sun burned but treated with the Aquaphor and vitamin E. I met other cancer patients during this phase of my journey that came from all different walks of life. One woman was a professor at Brown University. She didn't have children and wasn't married. Here was this brilliant, beautiful lady all alone in a hospital johnny fighting for her life. It was such a dichotomy. I was a Childrens' Care Director in a gym 15 hours a week and she was an educator at a prestigious university clocking endless hours. I was a wife and mother of 3. She was single with no kids. I was intimidated by her intelligence initially.

I even felt beneath her because of her profession. Then I came to understand why Crayola makes such a big box of crayons. No 2 are the same, and neither are we as humans, thank God. We were both sitting in that waiting room for the same reason. We were united in our survivorship. Another lady was battling breast cancer for the 2nd time. This, of course, shook me to my core. I never wanted to hear those words Dr. Semine had uttered on May 4th, ever again. But, this lady did hear those words, again, and did her 2nd tour of duty with courage and prowess. I scheduled my appointments in the morning around the same time every day. I usually met up with my 2 new 'sisters' at least 3 days a week in the waiting room. It didn't take long to realize there were no egos there. We had different situational circumstances but all wanted the same outcome. One thing I actually looked forward to during Zap hour was my heated discussions with my radiation technician, John. He was flippin' fantastic with the exception of one major flaw in his character. He was a lifelong fucking Yankees fan! BOO. It was so much fun shooting the shit with him debating player's statistics, game calling, pitching duels, A-Rod/Varitek, pretty boy Jeter and his ridiculous batting stance, daily standings, and all the rivalry associated slurs. It was doubly fun when Susie was with me! The interaction with John before heading in for my daily boob beam was positively medicinal for my psyche. After the first 1 or 2 appointments the nerves had left the building but verbally sparring with John added some spike to the punch! He would accompany me in to the radiation room. He adjusted me on the cold table. Then he went behind his control window and ZAP. It literally took less than a minute. The only day I had off from radiation was Thanksgiving. Jules and Steve hosted that year and it was wonderful. I still wore a bandana, big earrings and extra make up. I was closing in on the big finish and was so thankful to be breaking bread with my family. I felt so happy that day but without skipping a beat I was back on the road to Rhode Island the next morning. I was given the option of taking that day off too, but I wanted to stay on track for a December 13th curtain closing. The next week, and I don't remember which day, elevated Dr. Tom to an even higher pedestal. As I stated he and I shared our love for the Red Sox. Most fans listened to WEEI sports radio to get their fix on everything sports. It hadn't occurred to me that Dr. Tom was one of the many listeners. I had signed up to be a WEEI insider online. This threw me in a pool of thousands to win random prizes either online or on the radio. One day, while driving myself to radiation, I was atypically listening down the dial on another station. I never strayed from 85.0 A.M but for reasons I can't recall (chemo brain), I didn't have it on that day. I arrived at my appointment early and Dr. Tom happened to catch me after I changed into runway worthy stylish johnny. Seriously, someone should design a more fashionable garment. This piece of puke blue tissue paper wasn't exactly a mood elevator. I didn't typically see him on beam days, only for my weekly checkups. He said he'd heard my name called out on the contest line of WEEI while he was in his office. He didn't hear me call in so HE tried to call my cell phone and my home phone. What doctor does this?! When I got home I emailed WEEI and explained that I was on route to radiation and missed my shout out. They sent me my prize anyway! I won a Nintendo 64 game for the boys! I never would've known if Dr. Tom didn't mention it to me or leave messages on my phones. He ultimately did so much more for me in my quest for insurance coverage too. December 13th finally arrived. Eric took the day off to take me to this last romp with radiation. The ladies I'd come to know, intimately, decided a future lunch was in order. One of my 'sisters' gave me a star ornament for our Christmas tree with HOPE engraved in it. I had told them that I had a special twinkling star guiding my way and she remembered. My star is Nana and she presents herself to me in many spiritual, virtual, and physical ways...even as of this writing. I decided to bake some treats for John and I packed them in a Red Sox tin! They were chocolate chip crescent rolls topped with confectioner's sugar. I was unusually elated giving them to him before my final beam of life. I hugged John and one of his assistants, changed back to my regular clothes, and practically skipped into Eric's open arms. He said 'you're done and I'm so proud of you. I love you, now let's go'. We got to the car and he had a beautifully wrapped gift waiting for me in the trunk. I had a collection of Willow Tree angels and he'd gotten me the Angel of Hope. My jaws and ears were in pain from smiling. My tear ducts were dry from crying. My heart was beating rapidly from excitement. I called the boys. I called Mom and Dad who were heading out to Julie's. I called Kenan. I called Susie. I called Lynn. I called Cara. I called Julie. Eric and I had decided we'd celebrate with a special lunch on route home. I knew my parents were visiting Julie and Steve that day in their new house. After a wonderful lunch we surprised them all to celebrate. And my first word on the phone when I reached everybody I called was...I'M DONE!

CHAPTER NINE

I could barely wait until Christmas. We celebrate with my side of the family every Christmas Eve, usually at my parent's. We each pick a 'special' person to buy or make gifts for. Cara and Billy couldn't make the trip that year and it turned out that Cara had picked me. She created a beautiful binder about my year with photos, poems, quotes, gestures and a gift certificate for an onboard credit toward a cruise we were taking with them and Lynn's family in February. I treasure it to this day. My niece Devyn had written an essay about me and Dad, during his traditional grace, toasted my victory over breast cancer. Right before dinner Kenan wanted us all to come to the front porch. Zack would be testing for his driver's license in January and had been saving for a car. He found a Chevy Nova through my brother and much to our surprise; Kenan had the Nova detailed and ready to roll for Zack that Christmas Eve. I, as a mom, had never seen Zack so deliriously happy. Eric and I, in turn, became just as delirious. It was just one of those moments when your kid's happiness instills happiness within you. It was one hell of a year for my boys and my brother capped it off with a bang. There is no earthly man ever created that is a step above Kenan. My boys cherish the ground he walks on. My sisters and I hold him in such reverence. My entire family, in laws and outlaws, hang on his every word. We'll never forget the gesture he made 12/24/2006 for Zack and believe me, there have been countless more. I really missed my nana that Christmas. I mean, I miss her every single day but THAT Christmas her physical absence was palpable. My Da had passed away in 1980 from prostate cancer and Nana continued to live with us. She would've been a captain on my team throughout my entire journey. She would've been best friends with Will Power. She was a beacon of light and positivity and her glass was always $\frac{1}{2}$ full. If the grass seemed greener on the other side of the fence she'd say to fertilize your own lawn better. She lived to 96 years old. She used to attribute this to Certo with grape juice, Geritol, and a shot of midday scotch! She ate ice cream every night, loved everything sweet, and quit smoking Parliaments in her 80's! Her skin was white as snow, silken and lustrous. I'm not sure she ever owned a razor because she never had to shave her legs! Her hair was pearly gray. Her favorite color was purple, same as mine. She loved to iron watching the ABC soaps. She rarely wore a dress but could rock a pantsuit like nobody's business! In 1999 we had a memorial service for her at the church by the sea. Nana showed up, at the end of the pew in a purple pantsuit, looking straight ahead at the altar. I noticed her first and thought maybe the heat was getting the better of me. I elbowed my brother and dad who both saw this vision. One by one my siblings and mom looked at her. After the mass I made a mad dash to find this handsome lady. Poof, she vanished. We all truly believe Nana showed up to her own service to let us know she was ok. When I got diagnosed with breast cancer I looked to the sky every night for comfort from her. A star began to twinkle at me one night when I was talking out loud to it. Now stars had always twinkled in the celestial twilight but this was different. Nana was reaching out to me. Another 'sign' from her was on a walk I was taking in the neighborhood one day during chemo. I passed these sidewalk flowers every time I walked by that never had caused a second thought. That day I was talking to Nana while approaching these flowers and a comforting breeze came out of nowhere. A gorgeous, fragrant scent whisked around my face like I'd never smelled. It was her. I got home and called Susie immediately because I knew she wouldn't consider me crazy. Susie's mom had passed away, suddenly, in 2003. She too believed in signs from our loved ones. That ambrosial bouquet was complete

111

confirmation that Nana was with me in spirit which fueled my fire even more. Today I have a tattoo on my left forearm in honor of her. It's a shooting faceted purple star with 'NANA' scripted as the tail. The irony in it is that she hated tattoos but she loved her grandchildren's independent spirits. She wouldn't like the idea of me having a tattoo, but she would love it because I do. Though missing Nana that Christmas Eve was difficult, we still had the same wonderful time we did every year. Dad concluded the evening with his reading of 'Twas the Night before Christmas' surrounded by his grandchildren. My hair was just beginning to come in but I still wore a scarf. I would begin my nightly dose of Tomoxifen the next week and New Year's was the around the corner...CHEERS.

Eric went to visit his dad in Fort Myers that January. I was so happy he did because he only saw my father in law a few times a year. While he was away I threw a celebration for myself at a restaurant in the next town. I wanted to share my elation and joy of triumph over breast cancer with Susie, Lynn, my mom, Julie and Shelby. Cara was in Pittsburgh but wouldn't have missed it had she been here. I had heard on WEEI that my favorite sports commentators, Mikey Adams and Pete Shephard were hosting their show from this place and I just knew it was where I should party! It was also the same restaurant Eric took me to for lunch when I completed radiation. Julie had secretly arranged for us to be seated at the best possible table, right in front of the WEEI set up. What a night it turned out to be!

Mikey put me LIVE, on the air! It was a call in radio show so listeners were calling in wishing me well. An anonymous caller even sent over a bottle of Moet champagne! Patrons of the restaurant were sending us rounds of drinks and the owner truly hooked us up. It was also the 1st night my mom saw me without headwear! I proudly showed off my whiffle and I loved it! I wore a swanky silk sleeveless camisole, tight jeans, flashy earrings, and splashy make up to compliment my hair. We enjoyed illegal amounts of laughter over dinner. It is one of my favorite memories to date. It was now 2007. It was time to get back to work, and for new beginnings. It was time to give back. RELAY!

CHAPTER TEN

I had returned to work at the gym in January, both as Child Care Director and to resume my routine exercise program. I'd only lost a total of 9 pounds since beginning treatment. I wanted to gain about 7 of that back, in a healthy way, to weigh in at 125 pounds, a comfortable weight for me. I enlisted the help of George, the gym's owner and personal trainer. He was kind enough to train Eric and me for free as a perk of working at the gym. I settled in with ease, to my job in the kids' room. All the moms and dads were beyond gracious in welcoming me back. I had to answer a million questions about my health, treatment, side effects and other breast cancer related topics but I was happy to do so. I was elated to resume my normal schedule and obtain optimal health. Now, after I completed radiation therapy another battle was underway. Insurance wasn't covering the $30,000.00 radiation therapy expenses. Two years, two external reviews, a patient advocacy attorney, Dr. Tom, piles of paper trails and a news anchor's help later I won my case. We were now in serious debt having lived on credit cards with ludicrous interest rates for 6 months. We forged another battle with fury however, and came out on top. How can these companies continue to get away with this stress inducing nonsense? I was denied coverage of breast cancer radiation treatment because the insurance coding lists my type of therapy as not medically necessary and an investigative procedure...BULLSHIT. There was nothing 'investigational' about it. I had a cancerous tumor on my right breast near my chest wall which was surgically removed. I was then served a 6 month diet of chemicals to eradicate any surrounding cells that may have been compromised by little Bin. The next step in this program was to endure 7 weeks of radiation and then 5 years of estrogen blocking medication. Everything about the radiation was 'medically' necessary and nothing about it was 'investigational'. Boy did that piss me off. I remember telling my advocacy attorney that I wanted to tell my story on the news. She wisely advised me to avoid that at all costs because I could aggravate my review process. We were gloriously happy to put that baby to rest and attempt to put a few eggs back in our little nest. We're still attempting that, but are also LIVING life. Anything can happen to anyone at any time. While I'm alive, I'm going to respect my life by LIVING it! February was approaching fast and we had a cruise to get ready for! We went on that cruise, out of New Orleans, in the aftermath of Katrina. We were with the Stapletons and the Blumenscheins for the beginning of mardi gras. THAT was eye opening! Lynn's boys and ours couldn't get enough of the ladies flashing boobies for beads. The boys were mid-teens and giddily hormonal! This was another one of those questionable parenting moments but when my brother-in-law Billy disappeared for a while one afternoon and was discovered ogling with the boys, we decided we'd let it slide and chalk it up to a fun memory! The ship sailed for a week through the western Caribbean

118

and we had a blast. It was just what the doctor ordered and this time the doctor was me!

I decided to attend the initial meeting for the 2007 Mansfield Relay for Life committee volunteers when we got back from vacation. There were a few familiar faces and a lot of unfamiliar ones. Normally I'd be a nervous nelly in this situation, but I was so excited to participate that the nerves settled themselves. I listened to Kara, the committee chairwoman for 2007; speak about where help was most needed. The Survivor's Dinner was right up my alley. I had a few connections in terms of catering and the creative juices were surging. I signed up without hesitation. I couldn't wait to get out of the gate. The townspeople had poured their giving hearts out to our family and I hungered to pour back. I wrote a Thank You editorial in the local paper the week before Christmas but I knew since listening to Jon's speech in 2006 and attending the Relay that I had to be involved in some capacity. Eric and I joined Lifesavers, Jon's Relay team, as did my sister Julie. I got to work on the Survivor's Dinner, reaching out to restaurant and bakery owners, radio stations, my boys' karate studio, online networking and more. I felt reborn. I felt excited. I felt worth something. I felt needed. I felt ALIVE. Along with being a committee member I was also participating in the Relay on team Lifesavers which required fundraising. The American Cancer Society provides each participant of the Relay a page, online, to support fundraising efforts. I designed mine immediately after signing up, wrote a little blurb about my reason for relaying and sent it to everyone in my contact list, and Eric's. The response was ridiculous, in a spectacular way! Donations were coming in almost every day. Again, people got out of their own way to pay it forward, sometimes without ever having met me. The next meeting called 'Captain's Night' was in March where the captains of the Relay teams brought their team member lists and participation fees. I wasn't a captain but I attended out of curiosity. That meeting turned my life around and ultimately changed my whole purpose for being on this earth. Kara and the other committee members decided to ask me to be the 2007 keynote speaker! She told me to think about it and get back to her within a week or so. I never found the feather that knocked me over. After crying for about 5 minutes and talking about it to Jen (Jon's wife and Lifesaver captain) I gave Kara a resounding YES! I know in my heart that Jen had suggested me and I'll be grateful to her forever. I always sucked at public speaking, always. The few times I had to give oral reports in college I pretended I was someone else. I hated it. This would be different. I had something, a lot of things, to say. I couldn't wait to get home from the meeting to tell Eric. I often felt during our marriage that there wasn't much for him to be proud of me for. I mean I know I was, and am, a good mom. I guess in the career spectrum I didn't amount to much. I chose part time jobs to be home with my boys over a full time job. I believe whatever works for anyone's family is how they should play it. Full time wouldn't have worked for me or my personality. I didn't want someone else spending my time with my kids. Obviously there are situations that require 40 hour (or more) work weeks whether it's a single parent trying to make ends meet or a successful career path or just a personal choice. I don't feel like we made any 'sacrifices' to be home, as you hear some people say, except financially. But, Eric worked with many career oriented women and there were times I felt like I didn't measure up. I often felt this inferiority with my friends, and even sisters, who worked full time too but I never questioned our decision. I just butt sled down a few emotional black diamonds, dusted the powder off, and got right back on the slope! This speech would be my shining moment. I got home, told Eric,

123

cried again, and he beamed with excitement and pride. It was a great juncture in my life. It was truly a turning point that would circle around June at the Relay. I had about 2 months to prepare a seven minute speech. Initially I thought it'd be difficult to fill the time. As I immersed myself in writing I realized the opposite! I desperately wanted to motivate and inspire the relay participants. I also wanted to convey my message of urgency with regard to funding for this global epidemic. I spent hours selecting my words carefully and poured over quotes I found online. There was also this essential longing to make my boys, parents, husband, friends and family proud. As the spring garnered us with some choice weather days, we took the opportunity to get our 'just desserts' for fundraising. Troy would sell ice cream at the end of our street and donate every cent to the Relay. The donations filtered through my page on Lifesavers and helped our team become one of the top 5 fundraising teams for 2007! This was another gift our family received from my diagnosis. Our boys have taken the philanthropic helm and have captained many fundraising vessels, as many cancer families do. My nieces raised money through lemonade stands. My brother and niece swam a mile in a bay on Cape Cod to fundraise. It effortlessly became a family effort. Another springtime growth was my new Shirley Temple 'do'. Cancer survivors I've encountered had the same experience I did when my hair began to come in. When you think about it, it's like baby hair. It's virgin hair because the roots of the pre-treatment hair have been killed at their cellular level. It's all new! I know some who's have grown in gray. Some have had it grow in its natural tone and texture. Others had it grow in like when they were an infant. That was me! I was 45 with a mass of curls taking over my melon! I couldn't stand it at first but as it got longer, I began having fun with it. I swore off bandanas but found new ways to make it look vaguely stylish. My mom loved it! I couldn't wait for my eyelashes and eyebrows to grow in, and they did. In fact, so did a chin hair or two...what the fuck? Luckily they grew and disappeared into unwanted hair land but for a while I felt like I could've blended in very well at Hogwarts! The pubes were a different story all together. Talk about a fucking scratch soiree! I was so damn itchy as the hair grew in I could've used a fork down there! Unfortunately, my mock brazilizian wax, which occurred naturally via chemicals, was never put to good use in 6 months. Ladies, I just don't get it. When I was showering or in front of the mirror I felt like my 2nd grade vagina was staring back at me. For real, how does this make a guy horny? Or, for that matter, how does it initiate any sort of eroticism in a woman? It only made me more self-conscious than I was already. Eric never once paid any extra attention to my lady bits while it resembled a 7 year olds anatomy, so I never encouraged it. We have a double shower so there are times we conserve water and scrub up together...nothing. Not that I minded. The hotter the shower the hotter Eric and I just got dizzy from the heated moisture. Just to be clear, not my moisture, the showers! Yoga was all the action I needed. If you haven't tried it yet, do. I mean, DO! Twelve sessions and your pelvis will be penning you thank you notes! For the hair on my head I made a promise to myself when it began to grow in that I'd cut it as soon as it hit 8 inches from the nape of my neck. Wigs were never in the picture for me, but they are for many and donating my hair was something totally doable so why wouldn't I? I donated my 1st ponytail to Pantene Beautiful Lengths in 2011 and my 2nd in 2013. The 1st time took 4 years to grow that long because of the simple nature of it. Think of a 4 year old girl cutting her hair for the 1st time. It's usually shoulder blade length. The 2nd time only took about a year and a half to grow the 8 inch ponytail. I'm told by my hairdresser, Mr. Tabulous, that hair grows 1/2" a month on average. That seemed about right in my case. Zack and Troy have both donated ponytails too. Clay made a valiant attempt but decided to put his philanthropic efforts to other use, which he's done in sweet, harmonious, musical ways. Eric simply doesn't have the hair. Sorry honey!

CHAPTER ELEVEN

March, April and May of 2007 were very busy months. I immersed myself at work, karate, scorekeeping baseball, Relay initiatives and fundraising. I reconnected with local restaurants and bakeries to confirm their interest in the 2007 Relay. I also contacted WEEI, via email, for some shout outs on their program. Let's face it. Relay for Life is in most states. I wanted to get our town of Mansfield on the radar. I arrogantly thought that since Mikey Adams and Pete Shephard had been standouts in my post treatment celebration, it'd be no problem to give my team some air play for the Relay. I'm also a huge fan of Larry Johnson's cartoons. I'm not sure how it universally connected, but WEEI did give me a blip. I just chalked it up to karma and a little obnoxious persistence on my part. Mr. Johnson is a cancer survivor himself. He was the one who answered my emails and suggested other ways to promote my cause. Jules and Steve hosted Easter (as they do most years because it's usually close to the twins' birthday). They came up with a fun activity for everyone to tie dye t-shirts in my honor for the Relay. All of them had to say 'In it to win it' somewhere on the shirt. I had recited this phrase at nauseam to my family so they decided to run with it. A shirt was made for everyone. This said to me that all of my family planned to be at the 2007 Relay for Life to support me as the keynote speaker (with Blumenscheins excused).

Julie was a Lifesaver so she was committed to being there but I didn't know who else would show up. We all spent the afternoon coloring luminaria bags, which sold for $5 each, benefitting the Relay. Every single bag at Julie and Steve's was dedicated to me, while raising money too. The money was terrific. The messages and pictures, however, were priceless. They have a special place in my hope chest today. June was fast approaching and I needed to grow a pair. The Sun Chronicle newspaper did a feature article on me the week of the Relay, as they do with every keynote speaker. Our local paper included me in its coverage of the upcoming Relay. News was certainly buzzing that I'd be kicking off the event. I had to speak, very publically, and I had an opportunity to truly make a difference. I could impart my views on everyone in attendance as well as the media audience. I could also make a difference in myself...WITHOUT FURTHER ADO.

I needed to be at the Mansfield High School early due to my committee responsibilities. My speech was on index cards in my back pocket. If I lost even one of the cards I was up shit's creek, with NO paddles! I checked in with Amy, the dinner coordinator, who appeared extremely relaxed. I introduced a new contributor to the Relay and I wanted to insure a smooth outcome. My neighbor's sister owned a restaurant with her husband in the next town. They agreed to supply our Relay with a generous portion of the Survivor's Dinner. It was wonderful. Enlargements of previous Relay photos were displayed around the high school cafeteria and a solo guitarist I booked was setting up. The music was a first for the dinner so I patted myself on the back for making it happen. I allowed myself to be proud that night, of myself. Everything seemed to be going off without a hitch, except the butterfly party kicking it in my stomach. I was thoroughly prepared but was acutely aware of the ticking clock. As the minute hand edged closer to 6:00 p.m, I edged closer to hysteria! I left the cafeteria to head out to the track. I wanted to confirm where Eric, Zack, Clay and Troy would be standing to insure eye contact. The track and the soccer field at Mansfield High School were packed. I was trying not to take a clonazepam, my anxiety medication, to overcome my fear of public speaking. Zack would say, so far so good to this point. I did feel nervous but I kept telling myself the nerves were normal, similar to a prospective actress auditioning for a role or anyone who has ever experienced a trying job interview. I found my family. I found my parents, siblings and their families. My aunt Brenda made the trip from Marshfield to see me speak and Carol, my mother in law, came too. Lynn broke speed limits to get there from work and Susie, who had told me she wouldn't be able to make it, changed her plans and surprised me on the field. Having Lynn and Susie there was a saving grace. If they hadn't made it, I would've felt like an apple pie at Thanksgiving with 2 slices missing before it was served. It just wouldn't have been the same. I can't count the number of friends, neighbors and townspeople who wished me good luck. Wendy, who I'd become closer with and is a sister Survivor, was there,

135

celebrating almost 8 years of her breasts free of cancer. Her story as it relates to her and her sisters is nothing short of amazing. Wendy is not only a survivor but a giver, an anonymous volunteer, a confidante, and a trusted, generous friend. Her family and ours went on to enjoy many Survivor Dinners together. I gave my dad a sneak peak of the speech, more for my own reassurance than his curiosity, and he said 'Way to go honey'. One of the committee members came to get me right at that moment, thank God because the floodgates were about to open and surge! When any of us Connell girls get positive reinforcement from our dad the tears are inevitable. That's why we're referred to as the Crying Connells! I headed up to the bleachers that overlook the track to listen to the chairwomen welcome everyone. Then Katie, our American Cancer Society representative spoke statistics about cancer and about where the Relay money is directed. When Katie concluded her speech it was my turn. It was a very sunny evening so I was wearing sunglasses. My rotini hair was held back by a headband. I wore my new Survivor t-shirt instead of my Committee one. I scanned the enormous crowd one more time, heard Kara introduce me and almost completely freaked out. For a split second I thought that I needed to find some inconspicuous way out of there. What the fuck did I get myself into? Who did I think I was and why would this huge audience engage in anything I had to say? That second ended and it was...SHOWTIME.

I did some yoga breaths, glanced at my index cards, and then realized the loud applause that was welcoming me. This, of course was both relieving and scary. When the applause ended you could hear a q-tip hit the ground. It was now up to me to fill the Mansfield track with an informative, entertaining, attention grabbing 7 minutes. I had months to prepare for this moment but was I really prepared, to strip down and tell my story? YES!

CHAPTER TWELVE

'Welcome everyone! My name is Noreen Taranto and I'm a breast cancer survivor.' I had to consciously look away from my parents or I'd be unable to continue. My mom had caught my eye which caused me to tear up. I temporarily lost my vision, unable to see my index cards. Everything was a complete blur...uh oh. Luckily, clarity set in quite quickly, unlike other times in the past when anxiety reared its ugly head. I looked instead, at the 'HOPE' outline of luminaria bags that were yet to be lit on the bleachers across the field from me. Although a sea of humans was within my immediate perspective, I projected my voice and sight slightly above their heads. It was just easier that way. After an initial throat clearing, the confidence and composure snow balled as I spoke. My momentum gained stride with each word. I was in my element, finally. I was a little ripple that could make some big waves! I conveyed my belief that cancer doesn't target any specific culture, race, sex or age group. It just pulls back the arrow and shoots. We are all unknowing targets. I shared my personal story, from my clean mammogram, subsequent MRI, diagnosis, treatment, and how I involuntarily joined the world wide club known as cancer Survivors. Our government needed, as it does today, a lesson in follow through and integrity. There have been many promises about funding for cancer that haven't been fulfilled. I amplified my opinion to this captive audience that we must use the technology available to us. The cliché is that you can drive a horse to water but you can't make him drink. Well, we can certainly pour salt on him to make him thirsty. I called on everyone at the Relay to salt our elected officials. Salt them with phone calls, emails, voice mails, letters, protests or whatever it takes to get the requisite funding that cancer beckons and its patients deserve. Then I told my attentive crowd a story. My parents had an apple tree in their yard that Eric and I had given them when it was a sapling. The tree bloomed with ripe apples and grew to overshadow their driveway. While I was in the process of writing my speech I often thought of this special tree. Then the light bulb went off and I knew why. It reminded me of me, and every other cancer patient. An initial seed is planted. A tree grows with the proper care. The apples blossom over time. These apples have tough skin protecting their inner meaty layers and core, as do we. When cancer 'picks' us, like an apple is picked off of a tree, our thick skin is challenged. Our inner selves are vulnerable and we are shaken to our core. I chose to plant another seed and let it grow, and I have grown so much. I disclosed how difficult this experience was on my family but how we left negativity at the door and no matter how hard it knocked, we never let it in. I never, ever asked 'why me'. That, to me, is pointless. Instead I would tell my boys or anyone who wanted to engage me 'why not me'. I'm a small minnow swimming in life's big ocean. Cancer can target anyone so why not land it's hook in me? The rest of the speech was filled with gratitude toward our community, my euphoria on being a committee member, ideas on awareness, and a closing statement dedicated solely to Zack, Clay, Troy and Eric. I turned into a Crying Connell again, but was able to curb the amount of weeping. Since each of my boys was a baby I've kissed them goodnight with 5 special kisses, LOVE, PEACE, STRENGTH, HOPE, COURAGE. I decided to blow these special kisses to them from the podium symbolizing saying goodnight to the breast cancer. Then I told Eric I loved him in front of the town of Mansfield. I thanked him for digging me out of the trenches when I fell in too deep. And I told him how thankful I was for that fateful day, May 4th, 1984 that he was hanging on the steps of the campus center at UMass and it was game over. Interesting, isn't it? May 4th brought Eric into my life then 22 years later it brought me my diagnosis. I hated learning I had breast cancer on May 4th, 2006 but looking in the rearview mirror I consider it a windfall that gusted into my life and changed my whole direction, just as Eric did in 1984. I concluded with my appreciation toward everyone in attendance and then officially kicked off Relay for Life, Mansfield, 2007! WALK ON...

I barely made it to the track before my sister Julie enveloped me in a huge bear hug. She and I were both crying and my baby sister then kissed me and told me how proud she was of me. Then my brother, Shelby, Shea and Devyn presented me with a bouquet of the most gorgeous pink roses I've ever laid eyes on. I made my way through my parents, aunt, and mother in law, Susie, Lynn and a host of other well-wishers before I connected with my boys and Eric. It was vehemently important that I made them proud. Each of them told me, I did. The first lap of each relay is called the Survivor's Lap. I blended in with the rest of the survivors and their families with all of my family wearing the 'in it to win it' t-shirts they had made on Easter. I felt like I was walking on air. After the Survivor's Lap all of the survivors and guests were invited into the high school for the Survivor's Dinner. It honestly felt like we were royalty. I'm not sure if I even ate any of the food I helped to organize because of the buzz around me. My mom was in her glory seeing me garner all this attention. People were congratulating me, the boys, Eric, my parents and my family on

145

the success of my speech. It went on to be a wonderfully emotional, meaningful and memorable night. I embraced my newfound identity as an advocate for breast cancer. My voice was heard, but I had so much more to say and do. The rest of that summer was spent at karate where Zack received his 3rd degree black belt and Troy received his 1st degree black belt, watching Red Sox games, going to the beach and all the summer stuff that families do. I was still working at the gym when school resumed. Another fitness center in town made me an interesting offer that ultimately caused me to switch jobs. I transitioned to a Child Care Supervisor, soccer tots coach and event planner. Many of the parents I'd known at the 1st gym came to the new place too. It was great because I knew a lot of the members and their kids. It turned out especially great because I met one of my best friends there. Debbie was, and is, a school bus driver in our town. During the few hours she had free in the mornings, she'd oversee the kids' room with me. She'd been doing the job already, and when I came onboard we immediately clicked. Debbie's mom is a breast cancer survivor. Deb has supported me in all my efforts and takes a keen interest in my advocacy. We got through fall and winter of 2007 celebrating all the holidays and enjoying family time. Then in March of 2008 another piece of shit hit the fan. CRAP...

CHAPTER THIRTEEN

March 18, 2008.
'First, I'm fine, but I have another
procedure to endure next week. I got the
pathology results this morning from a
'punch biopsy' I had done a few weeks
back. This was a lesion that I found, had
checked by my oncologist and
dermatologist. They both concurred I
should consult my breast surgeon. After
the biopsy, it was subsequently sent to a
Specialized Melanoma lab. It was
confirmed that the lesion is compound
dysplastic nevus with abnormal/severe
atypia. This means, in laymen's terms, that
I caught the horse before it got out of the
barn and ran a really bad race. Compound is

one of 3 ways to describe the stage of the growth... Dysplasia means precancerous AND a change in cells or tissue. Nevus is the growth itself. The procedure next Thursday is to remove more surrounding tissue to assure the doctor (and me) of clear margins. Please, please, please don't worry about this and know that I'm very optimistic. And also, DO NOT associate this with my breast cancer. This was on my left nipple, but is in the skin cancer family...totally different. I wanted to make all of you aware of this before Sunday. I want to have a great day and holding information in is getting old for me! Well, that's the scoop.'

This was an excerpt of an email I sent to my family the week before Easter. Julie and Steve were hosting again. I knew I'd be a little off and could guarantee when I saw my dad, if I didn't disclose what was happening I'd lose it. I preferred to let them in ahead of time. I had noticed a funky purplish mole shaped mark on my left nipple in February. I watched it, obsessively, for a couple of weeks. It was growing. I didn't like the looks of it so I saw my dermatologist. He didn't like the looks of it either. He referred me to my oncologist, who also didn't like the looks of it. I questioned Dr. Browne about melanoma and how in the world would it grow on my nipple. The only time my boobs saw the sun was one day on Martha's Vineyard when Eric and I were dating. We went to Gay Head where clothing was optional and I was feeling free spirited. Those pictures are tucked securely away! Dr. Browne informed me that melanoma can grow and spread to any part of the body.

She's even seen it inside a patient's vagina. WHAT? She referred me to my breast surgeon who agreed with everyone else. Dr. Partridge took a skin sample from the interior of the mark and sent it to pathology. Needless to say I was a super-sized bundle of nerves. Dr. Partridge called me a couple of days after the punch biopsy to inform me that the local pathologist requested the sample be sent to a specialized melanoma lab in the south. She needed my permission. I was shitting pickles. After another few days of thread hanging I received a call from Dr. Partridge at work. The mark was basically pre melanoma and she strongly advised me to have more tissue removed to affirm clear margins. Debbie was with me when I got the call, thank God. She went and found Eric, who was working out. I almost puked.

We all regrouped. Deb and I continued
playing with the kids until our morning shift
was over. I, again, convinced myself not to
worry unless there was something to worry
about. Another great Easter was had by all
and the twins enjoyed another wonderful
birthday. They were now 7. My dad was
inquisitive about the email I had sent to
everyone but knew I didn't want to make a
big deal out of it. He pulled me aside, put
both of his hands on my arms, looked me
dead in the eyes and asked if I was
absolutely positive this had nothing to do
with my breast cancer. I reassured him it
didn't. I couldn't tell him, however, that I
was completely in the clear. I had to have
the minor procedure, wait on the results
and go from there. Eric took me to the
slice and dice of my areola. It went off
without a hitch and minimal pain. The pain

was of the ass kind! It was a pain in the ass to play the waiting game once again, but, no chickens had hatched yet so why start counting? Dr. Partridge called me the following week with the good news that the surrounding tissue of the growth showed clear margins. She also commended me for being vigilant. Ever since my diagnosis and treatment I'm extremely in tune with body. I listen to it and if it tells me something is out of whack or suspect, I have no qualms about seeing the appropriate physician. Some may call this over cautious or even paranoid but I don't give a flying rat's ass. I learned my lesson from putting off that breast MRI in 2006. If my body is reaching out to me with the language of pain, swelling, numbness, or anything unusual I pay close attention. It was during that year that my genitalia began speaking to me, loud and clear. Sex had become extremely painful. I initially attributed it to the chemo induced menopause leaving my vagina dry as dust. I've come to discover that many female chemo patients experience these symptoms but suffer in silence. I did the same. Eric and I would be fooling around and he, sadly, thought the moans I emoted were derived from passion. He thought my hands pressed so firmly on the wall above my head were from the throws of wild sexual pleasure. Not. I was in complete unmitigated agony. His thrusting felt like he was sandpapering my hooch with shards of broken glass. And, to protect his ego and his bravado, I kept up this charade for quite some time. Then I couldn't bear the physical pain anymore. I had to tell Eric what was going on and hope for his support. We agreed that I should

check in with Dr. Jill. She recognized that
I presented inflammation and parch
overload. During this exam I also told Dr.
Jill about the pre-melanoma on my areola.
She brought up my chart and carefully read
through what had happened. She then
asked me if I ate a lot of red meat. At
that time my favorite 'go to' meal was steak
and fries. I was also a huge cheeseburger
junkie. Dr. Jill suggested I give up the red
meat due to the hormones the animals are
fed. Why wouldn't I? DONE. It's been 5
years red meat free for me!   She sent me
to my obstetrician who prescribed an
estrogen cream (which I cleared with my
oncologist) citing that it'd be like watering
only the part of the lawn that needed it. I
was concerned because my tumor was
estrogen fed and I didn't want to feed any
other cells that may be bandying about. My

ob/gyn also referred me to a specialist, prominent in everything vagina! After months and months of creams, steroids, vaginal suppositories, tubes of lube and appointments my specialist recommended me to a pelvic floor physical therapist. Now, I'd been to PT before, for my knee and back but my vagina? I'd never heard of such a thing. I did my research and became hopeful that this new regimen may help me to heal. I was swimming in guilt for such a long time that I couldn't be the exciting, passionate partner Eric deserved. I felt constantly chafed, like those Indian sunburns we used to give each other in grade school, except this wasn't on my arm! I began the PT at some point in 2009. My therapist, Raquel, confided in me that a large percentage of her practice were breast cancer survivors. Some women are fortunate to see their periods return post treatment. I was thrown head first into menopause at 44 and today, at 51 am still riding the wave. Raquel taught me exercises to practice at home and provided me with dilators of varying sizes. Eric was supposed to help me with my homework, which didn't happen often enough. I didn't understand it. Why wouldn't he want to help me as much as he could? It would only benefit him. Our private time, as is with many couples, was extremely limited when the boys were around. Zack had begun his college career at Kent State University in the fall of 2008 so he wasn't home throughout the school year but Clay and Troy were, and our rooms are all on the same floor. I think Eric was being cautious, and the homework assigned could be a turn on. I don't think he wanted to start something I couldn't finish! I continued with Raquel, for my own well-being and Eric's. One day she asked me if I'd be interested in speaking alongside her at the Dana Farber Institute in Boston, MA. She was giving a seminar on the benefits of pelvic floor therapy with sidebars on how it relates to cancer patients. Just like when I was asked to be the keynote speaker at the Relay, I couldn't answer 'Yes' quick enough! Her specific type of treatment was finally helping me and I was beginning to feel somewhat feminine again. I met Raquel at the acclaimed facility one Tuesday night. After she presented her information it was my turn. I was so happy to speak about this highly personal issue because for so, so many its considered taboo. It was another accomplishment for me that never would've happened had I not had breast cancer. I spoke about my arid, inflamed vagina in front of Dana Farber clinicians! Are you kidding me? Wonders truly never will cease! This was after a summer that I became ornery and defensive. I was irresponsible with regards to alcohol. I'm fairly confident today that I had developed PTSD. I was overtly strong from the moment I was bitten by the cancer fangs, through surgery, chemo and radiation. I really never let myself purge. The summer of 2009 I began to atypically have a martini while making dinner, every night. I turned a blind eye to the interaction of my clonazepam and alcohol. I accused Eric of controlling and smothering me. I pumped the mood swings back and forth and would escape what I thought were the confines of my house whenever I could. I needed to

159

see Dr. Jill again, just to talk. After explaining my unflattering and possibly dangerous habits to her, she implored me to either have a drink OR take my medicine. I obviously couldn't do both. She encouraged me to continue my work out routine and to possibly seek counseling. Eric wasn't on the counseling band wagon so any type of marriage counseling wasn't an option. Our insurance didn't cover it anyway. I decided to take things into my own hands. I amped up my exercise routine, began vigorously walking, and made a valiant attempt to use my dilators. The autumn leaves were coloring our woods. It was my favorite time of year. Then, a conversation I had at the gym with a friend of mine changed everything. That conversation became the next turning point for me sending me off to a new and long awaited direction. I wanted to participate in a particular event for a few years but always said 'next year'. Well, Jules, my flawlessly beautiful friend convinced me to register with her and 'next year' became 'this year'. We'd be walking and tent buddies for the Susan G. Komen 60 mile 3Day. We had 8 months to train and raise the requisite $2300.00 each. I couldn't wait to pound the pavement! I didn't know how much this would impact me, on a personal level. I CAN WALK FOR MILES AND MILES AND MILES...

CHAPTER FOURTEEN

I met Jules when I watched her daughter in the kids' room at the gym. Jules was the stunning beauty I would always bump into when I looked like something the cat dragged in. She could've walked off of the cover of Vogue when I saw her anytime, anywhere. It got to be annoying! Her oldest daughter and Troy are the same grade so she and I volunteered in their classes together. I encountered her on the baseball field countless times when I was scorekeeping in my baseball garb and she was channeling a Sports Illustrated Model. The black fly in the chardonnay is that Jules has a heart of gold and is genuinely nice. She is a loving mother of 4 and a hopelessly devoted wife. Her philanthropic efforts are immeasurable. I knew we'd make a good team if I could cloak my ever present self-consciousness! We did. We made a spectacular team. During the course of our training we held 5 fundraisers. Each one was different. We knew everyone would be out in full force in the spring of 2010 fundraising for the Relay. I remained on Lifesavers but told Jen and Jon that I needed to focus my energy on the SGK 3Day. Jules and I decided to start early. She hosted a Partylite Night in January to get the ball rolling. We went on to hold a Silent Art Auction in March, a Band Together Now concert and a Pub Crawl in May. Then my sister Cara held a Raise Your Glass for the Cure wine tasting event in her home in Pittsburgh that June. Eric and I jumped in

163

the car and took a road trip to surprise Cara and Billy for the weekend so we could be there. It was perfect. Their friends, neighbors and colleagues put Jules and I over the $16,000.00 mark! The events and our own fundraising endeavors resulted in almost $17,000.00 raised! At the outset of this decision to do the walk, Eric was concerned about my ability to raise the $2300.00 required to participate. I was extremely hurt. He sucked the air out of my balloon for months until I announced to him that the Silent Art Auction would be in his co-worker's honor. She had breast cancer and I wanted to support her, as did he. Suddenly he was onboard. I harbored resentment toward him until the floodgates opened one night and we cleared the air. He understood my feelings and realized he hadn't put enough faith in me. I, though it took a long while, understood his trepidation too. We were still in the weeds financially, with no clear path, and I was embarking on this major fundraising effort. I never doubted my competence but he did. We now both know that one didn't impact the other and he completely supports my life's goal to contribute to the END of breast cancer. Jules and I walked strong over 3 humid, hilly, hot days and slept through 2 rainy nights. It was great. We heard many gut wrenching stories and many heartwarming ones too. I walked because I could. I walked because my aunt couldn't. I walked to raise a lot of money. I walked to heighten awareness and to louden voices. I walked so others won't have to face the devastating financial burdens of being a cancer patient waging war with insurance companies. I walked so cancer no longer has legs. We saw some familiar faces along our 60 miles. My sister Julie trailed us from the starting point until she found us about 3 hours in on the first day. She left her executive position to find us, kicked off her professional heels when she did and walked with us for a bit, barefoot! She was wearing purple. Again, someone simply was paying it forward. Eric's cousin drove by us beeping his horn loud and proud and then Kerry, my girlfriend from high school surprised us on day 2. She had been parked in her sand chair waiting for us for 2 hours at a cheering stop. We stopped to take some pictures but had to motor on. I'll always remember her being there for us that day. She doused us with motivation and quenched us with laughter. Day 3 Jules and I had agreed to finish strong, no matter what. We were both bubbling with blisters and exhausted but inhaled adrenaline with breakfast and kicked it into gear. The weather was perfect. The route through Cambridge and Boston was evocative, uplifting, historical and energizing. The 3 miles of power walking to the finish along Carson's Beach in South Boston was sun soaked, breath taking (literally), and invigorating. The 3Day isn't a race but Jules and I had agreed to walk strong and finish stronger. She was walking in honor of a close friend battling breast cancer for the second time. She carried her friend's spirit on her shoulder the entire weekend. We were greeted by both of our families, our close friends and a cheering squad at the finish line. I was deliriously happy to see Eric and the boys awaiting me with open arms. They were so proud of me! Lynn was there too with our friend Kathy. Jules and I were blistered, tired, sweaty and pimpled with road rash. I felt more beautiful than ever. It was an accomplishment I'd been waiting my whole life to find and achieve. It was a weekend that changed my perspective forever. The Komen 3Day affirmed what I'd been trying to practice, LIVING. I made a decision that weekend to truly celebrate my 5 year survivorship the following year by travelling to Italy. It had been a dream destination for Eric and me and after hearing the stories I did over the course of 60 miles I was going, come hell or high water. Eric and I were sitting on our deck the day after I got home. I said to him "I'm going to Italy. I'd love you to come with me but if you don't, I'm still going." His thoughts immediately went to our financial status but he thankfully came around quickly. He wanted to go as much as I did. We had a year to plan it and save for it, and we did! The following year we celebrated 5 years cancer free in Barcelona and Italy with our lifelong friends from college. Dreams are for the making and ours came true. The cruise was magical, especially since a week prior to leaving I was hit head on by a drunk driver. I toured Italy in a boot on my ankle! I thought I could be in Italy in a boot, or I could be home in a boot. I chose Italy! At some point during 2011 my son Clay had uncovered those notes I had scribbled during Troy's flag football practice. Clay was a freshman in college paying some of his bills by playing lead guitar in a band he'd formed. Clay took my words, rearranged them musically with his band and released 'Just Listen' to YouTube and ITunes in January, 2012. Every penny earned from 'Just Listen', an anthem to breast cancer, is donated to awareness or research. And every penny counted is a penny that counts! 'Just Listen' is still trending today and all monies raised are filtered through Clay and awarded to a breast cancer cause. We continue to feed the cancer kitty and help it to purr.

Since being diagnosed my purpose for being here, on this planet, has introduced itself all over again. I look in the mirror every morning and wonder how I can make a difference in someone's life, even for a minute. This mode of pondering has brought me such joy, and as a result, brought joy to my family. Let's face it, when Mom's happy, everyone is happy. I don't know what tomorrow will bring, but I'm confident it will involve little gestures, anonymous efforts, or public outreach to combat the global epidemic of breast cancer. I live by a quote I wrote for my speech at the Relay, 'Sometimes you have to swim against the current to coast in with the tide'. It was definitely a trying journey but they say the journey IS the destination. It certainly was an interesting one filled with speed bumps along the way, being led in the wrong direction but finding my way back, meeting fellow journeymen and women of the future while holding on to those from the past, weathering all kinds of storms, fending off unwelcome invaders, taking in some beautiful sights, getting my 'feet wet,' finding shelter, and growing up along the way. My breast cancer journey had me climb many hills and delve into many valleys. There are countless trails to set out on and I will continue to explore as I venture down the next path. I have the utmost confidence I'll walk right into my dreams if I 'Just Listen'.

www.ingramcontent.com/pod-product-compliance
Lightning Source LLC
Chambersburg PA
CBHW070651290526
45790CB00001B/267